The Hormone
of Closeness

The Hormone of Closeness

The role of oxytocin in relationships

Kerstin Uvnäs Moberg

The Hormone of Closeness: the role of oxytocin in relationships

First published in Swedish as *Närhetens hormon* by Natur & Kultur 2009

This English edition first published by Pinter & Martin Ltd 2013

© 2009, 2013 Kerstin Uvnäs Moberg

ISBN 978-1-78066-045-5

British Library Cataloguing-in-Publication Data
A catalogue record for this book is available from the British Library.

Set in Minion

Translator Kicki Hansard
Illustrator Aire Iliste
Editor Debbie Kennett
Index Helen Bilton

Printed and bound in the UK by TJ International Ltd, Padstow, Cornwall

This book has been printed on paper that is sourced and harvested from sustainable forests and is FSC accredited.

Pinter & Martin Ltd
6 Effra Parade
London SW2 1PS

www.pinterandmartin.com

Contents

Introduction

To be touched and to experience physical closeness is a fundamental need for us humans, just like all mammals. At the very beginning of life, it can be a life-deciding factor and, later on, it can be what stands between a healthy life and a life with depression and physical illness. The need to be touched lasts throughout life. A person, whether a child or an adult, who daily expects and receives touch in the form of a loving hug, a warm hand or a friendly massage is likely to be happier, healthier and have a greater ability and willingness to communicate with others. Touch shows us that we are safe, that someone cares about us, and it especially tells us that we are valuable. But touch also provides profound neurophysiological influences which affect our behaviour and our emotions. That is what this book is about.

The model of closeness

According to the 'closeness model' presented in this book, closeness through touch, warmth and light pressure give rise to the stimulation of nerves in the skin, leading to increased social interaction but also well-being and an immediate calming and relaxing effect. Of course, all the other senses also contribute towards the beneficial effects. When the closeness ends, the well-being and calm gradually subside and, if gone for too long, are replaced by discomfort, anxiety and tension. During closeness there is a sense of well-being, calm and relaxation whilst during separation, worry and tension arise. In this way, for example, the small child and the parent or the couple in love are drawn to each other. Closeness also stimulates the body's own healing system.

In this closeness model, oxytocin has a key role. Oxytocin is a substance originally associated with childbirth and breastfeeding but which also belongs with touch, closeness and nutrition. Oxytocin has a more important and complicated role than previously thought because it is also involved in a number of different bodily and mental processes. This book is about exactly that; how oxytocin works like cement that helps create and maintain human relationships throughout our lives and in doing so plays a key role in human growth and health.

Furthermore, the closeness model is overarching or constantly underlying the biological and neurophysiological structural and explanatory model for human social interactions and intimate relationships. In the past, especially in areas such as psychology and stress research, the emphasis was on the active role of separation. It is known that this is associated with discomfort and with elevated levels of stress hormones, but the calming effect of closeness has never been included in the model of explanation. In the closeness model, the focus is on relationships and touch.

Background

In 1988, in collaboration with an American colleague, I organised a so called Wenner-Gren Symposium in Stockholm with the then sensational title 'Is there a neurobiology of love?' or, in Swedish, 'Finns det en kärlekens kemi eller neurobiologi?' A number of scientists, from anthropologists, biologists, zoologists to doctors and veterinarians, got together to discuss these issues. The symposium was very well received and the various elements came to be published in the journal *Psychoneuroendocrinology*.

It was during this meeting that I put forward for the first time the possibility that oxytocin was not just a mothering hormone, but it appeared to have a role in co-ordinating all types of interactions of a peaceful nature by creating positive emotions and also favourable psychological and physical effects such as a sense of calm, reduction of anxiety levels and stimulation of healing properties.

The reason why I was brave enough to suggest this was that I had worked for many years alongside graduate students and colleagues and had studied the effect of oxytocin and how oxytocin release could be activated. A collaboration with a group of midwives at the Karolinska Institute had shown that breastfeeding and motherhood was so much more than just the transfer of milk, and that appropriate physical and mental adaptations also occurred. The next step to assume that oxytocin could be a co-ordinating factor was not a huge leap. I then went on to do some research with my co-workers and some graduate students. We performed a variety of animal experiments to show that oxytocin could, indeed, give rise to these effects and that touch could cause oxytocin release and hence the oxytocin effects.

My thoughts and ideas around touch and oxytocin resulted in the writing of the book *The Oxytocin Factor – Tapping the Hormone of Calm, Love and Healing* in 2000. Since then, research into oxytocin and its effects, especially in regard to various relationships, has sprung up around the world. It is perhaps not a coincidence that many of those currently working with oxytocin were present at the meeting in Stockholm in 1988. One of the reasons why oxytocin is studied with such intensity is because it reduces anxiety, induces well-being and enhances social ability and this raises the possibility of developing drugs based on an entirely new principle, namely the oxytocin factor. The same applies to the ability of oxytocin to reduce pain, create calm and lower blood pressure, counteracting inflammation and stimulating healing processes. Others have gone further and studied the effect of oxytocin with regards to relationships and tried to understand why positive relationships have such a favourable effect on health.

When I wrote the Swedish edition of *The Hormone of Closeness* in 2009 the picture had become clearer because so many others were working with oxytocin and documenting its effects. I therefore felt it was time to summarise the current situation and to show how oxytocin works in different types of relationships.

Oxytocin lies 'low' in our brain, which means the effects produced by oxytocin are not immediately apparent, as they don't become conscious. It is, therefore, important to get to know oxytocin and its effects (and naturally its cousin, vasopressin which is more associated with aggression and stress) for us to be able to understand ourselves and others better and also perhaps to learn to handle oxytocin in a good way. It is perhaps particularly important today when we are subjected on a daily basis to frightening information about climate destruction, wars and other atrocities. It is easy to turn our emotions off in such situations and put our head in the sand and not take notice. When oxytocin is circulating, we become aware of our feelings and therefore we can also change ourselves.

The book's approach

We humans are highly developed mammals with the ability to think, anticipate and plan. Nevertheless, we still carry many of the same predispositions as our ancestors who lived 40,000 years ago, even though our lifestyle has changed significantly. Our brains have gradually evolved but large areas are unchanged and still function in the same manner as in the first humans. Chapter 1 describes what the relational conditions looked like for our early ancestors and how modern society today affects our ability to deal with this mammalian heritage.

The closeness model, with oxytocin as the necessary factor, does not exclude other explanations but includes and highlights many different theories related to human motivation and interaction, for example, learning theory and attachment theory. Chapter 2 provides a description of these theories.

Chapter 3 provides a basic description of the brain and the nervous system to give an understanding of how hormones, neurones and neurotransmitters interact and make us feel what we feel and do what we do.

The fourth chapter describes the book's prominent figure – oxytocin – in more detail. Here it is explained how it was discovered, where it is made, how it becomes activated in the body and the effects it generates.

What do we really know about the impact of oxytocin at the beginning of life and its influence on attachment? Chapter 5 describes how oxytocin plays a key role in childbirth and lactation, but also more generally in connection with closeness early on in life.

Chapter 6 describes how the role of oxytocin has been shown to be extremely important in our relationships and for our well-being throughout life.

Trust is one of the key ingredients for a good relationship. In Chapter 7, oxytocin's significance for trust is discussed and explained in detail.

Closeness makes us feel safe and secure and it makes us feel good. But food also has similar qualities. What happens when the availability of food is greater than the availability of closeness? Chapter 8 discusses how nutrition and closeness can easily be confused when there is a lack of one or the other.

Research indicates that closeness and physical touch provide major positive effects, which is something that has been overlooked in medicine and psychology. Chapter 9 looks at how closeness gives us longer and healthier lives.

Chapter 10 mentions areas where oxytocin will be used but also looks at the dangers of unwittingly using oxytocin to increase well-being, trust and ability for social interactions. The book concludes with a discussion about what this new knowledge of the significance of oxytocin will mean to society.

Happy reading!

1

Our mammalian heritage

The genes and predispositions of today's humans are almost identical to those of prehistoric humans and are adapted for life in small groups where closeness, keeping together and harmony are vitally important. It is, therefore, necessary to discuss how changes in our living conditions affect modern man's prospects for closeness and physical touch. What is the impact of the modern western lifestyle – with its views of the body and soul being separate – when it comes to satisfying the original need for closeness? Today, the ideal to a large extent is to 'be' someone rather than 'belonging' to something. To manage on your own has become a virtue instead of a forced necessity.

In our modern society, there is a strong reliance on the rational and the intellectual. We feel that we can control our lives and our well-being through conscious thought processes and common sense. But our lives are not governed only by our conscious and rational thoughts. Beyond these there is an innate knowledge that helps us deal with life, and in particular with our social relationships. These essentially instinctive abilities have a broader influence in the lives of other mammals compared to humans, but they are included as a part of our mammalian heritage and affect us more than we think.

How mammals take care of their young

A characteristic common to all mammals is that they give birth to live offspring and that the mothers produce milk to feed their young. The English word 'mammal' comes from the Latin word for milk glands, *mammae.*

All animal species have instinctive abilities which help them to survive. A particularly important one is the ability to take care of their young. In parallel with the ability to produce milk, mammals have developed sophisticated innate behaviour patterns and physical reaction patterns which enhance the mother's and the offspring's chances of survival during the critical and vulnerable periods during and following birth and when the offspring are young. These adaptations increase the ability for the species to survive.

These patterns and adaptations, also known as *maternal behaviours,* are expressed slightly differently in various mammals. Pigs and rats, which have many and very immature offspring, naturally differ from the mammalian mothers who give birth to only one or two offspring, who perhaps are able to stand on their own legs straight from birth. But in principle, maternal behaviour focuses specifically on giving the offspring food, closeness and nurture as well as safeguarding and protecting them. For this to happen, it is important that the mother quickly learns to recognise and attach to them, especially if the offspring can stand on their own legs and be mobile from early on. As a rule, it is the mothers who look after their offspring, but there are some species where the male mammals help out. This is particularly true for mammalian species that live in pairs.

Nutrition, closeness and care

Most mammalian mothers not only provide milk for their offspring, but they also lie very close to them to keep them warm and they clean and lick them. The offspring are warmed by the mother and this enables them to maintain their body temperature and relax. The cleaning and licking is not just to wash the offspring but also contributes, together with the warmth, to making the offspring feel good and to feel relaxed and secure. Furthermore, it stimulates the offspring's growth and development. The mother herself also becomes calm and feels good during lactation and from the closeness of her offspring – something that actually contributes towards her wanting to stay with them. If she leaves them, she actually becomes worried and wants to return to this closeness.

Unafraid, social and calm for life

Closeness early on in childhood is also of importance in the long term. If rat pups receive a lot of nurturing and closeness early on in life, they not only become calm at that time but also less afraid, more social and more stress-tolerant as adults. In addition, these female rats become better mothers to their own pups. There are also studies showing that mothers and newborn babies can be positively affected in the long term if they get close contact with each other early on in life – especially if it happens straight from birth. It is precisely this ability for interaction and the child's ability to handle stress that is improved. In other words, the short-term effects become permanent.

The vulnerable need protection

A mammalian mother not only provides closeness to her offspring, but she also protects them through various innate behaviours. Birthing and new mammal mothers and their offspring are naturally especially vulnerable to attacks from other animals. Mammals often build a nest or find a dark and secluded burrow to feed and care for their young, where it is difficult for potential enemies to enter. It can be vital to give birth hidden and preferably when it is dark. Even pigs in captivity try to create a small nest in the straw.

Before the birth, it is common for women to tidy up and

make things nice. They're 'nesting' by making sure their home is organised and safe. Despite living in modern surroundings, humans tend to give birth at night (if the birth takes its natural course), we prefer to be in familiar secluded surroundings and have peace and quiet around us. Often we don't want to be completely on our own but prefer to have competent and supportive people with us at birth. If the mother is supported by others, the chances are that the mother and the child will survive and get a good start in life. We also want to have our newborn baby with us as soon as it has been born.

Some herd animals protect the birthing females and their newborn by all birthing at the same time. This 'minimises' the risky period when the herd is particularly vulnerable. Traces of these ancient mammalian patterns are also present in humans. For example, ovulation and menstrual cycles often occur at the same time amongst fertile women who live together for a long period of time.

Potential enemies have no respect for newborn mammalian offspring, whether they are in a nest or standing on their own legs. In the fierce world of mammals, there may be enemies both outside of and within the species, even within the family. Therefore, mothers have developed a special vigilance and a will to defend. This maternal aggression is triggered when the offspring are in danger.

Maternal aggression is also expressed by humans. Almost every mother can turn into a tiger when she feels that her child is at risk. Many mothers, especially when the children are young, also become a little extra cautious and scrutinise any unfamiliar environment to ensure that there is no threat of danger.

To recognise and attach is vital to life

For a young mammal, which stands on its own legs, to be able to get food, protection and closeness from its mother, it is important that the mother and offspring know who the other is. Therefore, an invisible bond is created between them, whereby they quickly learn to recognise each other and prefer each other over others. In research with sheep and goats, it has been shown that the mother's ability to learn to recognise and bond to her offspring is greatest immediately after birth and then quickly subsides after 24 hours. When the mother has learnt to recognise her own offspring, this is the only one who will receive her food, care and protection.

The offspring activate their own recognition systems. Early lactation appears to be particularly important for the offspring to bond with their mothers. Again, it is the offspring of mammals that live in herds which very quickly learn to recognise their own mothers. This early identification is vital for the survival of lambs, for example, where it is crucial not to get lost and go to the wrong mother because it would not be welcome there. If it loses the connection with the ewe, it will be abandoned without food and will eventually die.

Most mammals use multiple senses to recognise and bond with their offspring, and the sense that dominates varies. The less developed a species is the more important is the sense of smell. Rats, for example, recognise each other mainly through smell but a ewe also identifies her lamb through smell. Rats in particular, but also many other mammals, communicate with each other via scent signals. Pigs use a lot of sounds when they communicate. By varying the frequency of its grunting, the sow can call her piglets and let them know about her milk let-down.

In more highly evolved species, sight comes first. For us humans, vision plays a particularly important part for us to recognise each other. We also naturally use our touch and hearing and it has recently been discovered that smell is also important for a mother and child to recognise each other and to bond. However, this is done not only through our normal olfactory system but also through an ancient communication system that transmits information via pheromones, tiny substances that are transported through the air.

It is not only the relationships between mammalian mothers and their offspring that are driven by unconscious and instinctive abilities but the same also holds true, for example, in animals that live in pairs or in packs. The animals feel good and become calm through closeness with each other; they protect each other and they recognise each other via the different senses, like smell, sight and hearing. This is true to some extent of us humans; we are also influenced by innate and unconscious forces in our relationships as couples, families and other groups.

These days it is easy to believe that we humans are not so dependent on our mammalian heritage. We receive so much conscious knowledge through school and society that the intuitive, innate knowledge is usually not needed – at least that's what we think. Giving birth usually takes place in the presence of skilled personnel under controlled circumstances in hospital. Paradoxically, birth is beginning to change and more traditional approaches are being adopted during labour and birth to take advantage of the intuitive, unconscious knowledge of our mammalian heritage.

Family and relatives are no longer as important as they used to be because society has taken over many of their functions. Our close relationships have gone through major changes and the group and village community has been replaced by the workplace. To some extent we can change attitudes and habits in the name of democracy and equality, but the original ancient response patterns, generated during the time when we lived as hunter-gatherers, can be difficult to manage and change, staying just below the surface and affecting us without our conscious knowledge. Our mammalian heritage and ancestral group responses and patterns play tricks on us if we're not aware of them, but they could be used more positively if we were to truly embrace them.

2

Closeness and attachment

Through the ages man has always thought and pondered about relationships and social patterns, as can be seen in the old stories and legends. Religious teachings gave the view that man was above other mammals, and relationships and family patterns were viewed as something given by God. The body and the soul were considered independent of each other and, as it was thought that the soul had higher value, the body was relegated to a hidden existence. This belief was long lasting within philosophy where the power of thought and reason was considered to distinguish humans.

It was only in the 1800s, when Charles Darwin's theories of evolution received a hearing, that the ground was laid for the possibility of a biological explanatory model for human behaviour. But it was to be a winding road. The Russian scientist Ivan Pavlov's research on salivary secretion in dogs was a breakthrough and introduced the behavioural or learning theory explanatory model. However, this approach was considered to be too mechanical. Other psychological theories, offering broader explanations of irrational emotions and relationships, began to gain ground. But yet again, these theories focused solely on man's psychological and mental processes, and did not consider that they might have a biological explanation.

Modern theories on behaviour and relationships

There is still strong resistance towards biological models when explaining human relationships. However, the results of modern neurobiological research are increasingly showing that biological mechanisms have a decisive influence on how we behave and relate to other humans. In this chapter, we look at this research and describe some of the theories which suggest that human relationships have a biological root. In many respects these theories are supported by the closeness model.

Ivan Pavlov and classical conditioning

A mother who has breastfed knows that the milk starts to flow when she is nursing her child. After a while, the milk will start flowing as the child cries and seems hungry and finally, it might flow just by looking at or thinking of the child. This shows that the let-down of milk has become a *conditioned response*.

One of the people who first described how you can condition some physiological effects was the Russian physiologist Ivan Pavlov (1849–1936), who lived in St Petersburg. Pavlov's studies included the production of saliva and gastric juices in dogs. When dogs eat food that tastes and smells good, they begin to secrete saliva and gastric juices. In his experiments, Pavlov rang a bell when the dogs were eating. After a while, he removed the food and it transpired that it was enough simply to sound the bell for the dogs' saliva and gastric juices to be excreted. The secretion had become a conditioned response to the sound of the ringing bell.

Pavlov also explained how the conditioned responses develop. When dogs eat, they activate sensory nerves that go from the oral cavity and gastrointestinal tract via the vagal nerve to the areas of the brain where the production of saliva and gastric juice is regulated. Unless these sensory nerves are activated by food when it passes through the body and 'touches' the insides of the gastrointestinal tract – and to some extent by the smell of the food – there will be no production of saliva and gastric juices. However, production of saliva and gastric juices can become a conditioned response to a simultaneous sound. When this occurs, it is sufficient to ring the bell to produce gastric juices. The sound has 'taken command' of the saliva and gastric juice production and the original activation through the sensory nerves in the gastrointestinal tract is no longer needed.

Konrad Lorenz and imprinting

A certain type of direct learning, a kind of primitive form of attachment in some birds, was discovered by the ethologist Konrad Lorenz (1903–1989). He called the concept *imprinting*. He demonstrated how a newly hatched gosling immediately stores the image of the individual it first sees, and then follows it during a long period in its life. Interestingly, it doesn't have to be the mother goose or even a different goose that it imprints on and follows, but it could just as well be a human. Imprinting is an immediate form of learning, which under normal circumstances has a significant survival value for the newly hatched chicks.

Bonding

The concept of imprinting does not apply in the case of mammals. Instead, the word bonding has been used to describe the strong connection that occurs between female mammals and their offspring if they remain close to each other in the neonatal period. It was a long time before the existence of a variation of imprinting in humans was accepted. The American paediatrician Marshall Klaus was the first person to describe how mothers and babies seem to link to each other in a powerful way if they are close to each other after the birth. He coined the term bonding to describe the concept of a mother who is bound to her child.

In mammals the word bonding is used to describe the way that the mother recognises and accepts her own offspring. In sheep, for example, the ewe recognises her lamb and prefers it to others, and the relationship is reciprocated. When the word bonding is used about humans, the concept includes not only the fact that the mother recognises her child and prefers it over others but also describes the motherly behaviour, such as looking into the baby's eyes and talking baby language. The same principle applies when describing the child's bonding with the mother, often called attachment. It is not just about recognising and preferring each other; the quality of interaction is also a component.

Harlow and the surrogate mothers

In the 1970s, the American psychologist Harry Harlow (1905–1981) published a number of ground-breaking scientific papers, in which he explained the importance of soft and warm contact for mammalian offspring when they are young. Harlow studied rhesus monkeys. He suspected that the mothers were not only important for their young to receive food, but also the closeness and contact with the soft and warm mother helped them to develop into secure and harmonious adult monkeys.

Harlow created an experimental model and replaced the real mothers with two kinds of 'surrogate mothers'. One device consisted of a steel wire dummy with a bottle, which provided the baby monkeys with milk. The second device consisted of a dummy covered with soft terry towelling. Behind the cloth, there was a light that radiated heat. In some of the experiments, the terrycloth dummy was also provided with a bottle. The baby monkeys could rub up against the dummy, sit close to it and cling to it and could in this way get 'closeness', touch and warmth.

It was discovered that the absence of the real mother was

of great importance for the development of the babies. The monkey babies that only had access to the steel wire dummy were unable to socialise normally with other monkeys as adults. In particular, their sexual behaviour was evasive and disrupted. If the females did get pregnant, by being more or less attacked by the male, they did not take care of their babies in a way that rhesus monkeys ordinarily would do. They did not care about them and even behaved brutally and aggressively towards them. However, the babies who had access to the woolly and warm terry towelling dummy seemed better prepared and were, as adults, able to be part of the group relatively trouble-free. They also looked after the babies they gave birth to.

But there was also a difference between the monkeys who were reared by their own mothers and those who were reared with the warm and soft surrogate mother. I, myself, had the pleasure of seeing a later generation of Harlow's monkeys in a zoological institution just outside of Washington.

When I arrived, all the monkeys were in a large enclosure and they could only be viewed through a fence. Behind the fence, three groups of monkeys lived together. I was told that the monkeys that had grown up with the wire dummy were more or less never seen. They were out of view before the first visitor reached the enclosure. The monkeys we could see were thus those who had either been with the warm, soft terrycloth dummy or their real mother.

But even between these groups, there was a difference. As soon as we got to the fence, half of the remaining monkeys disappeared with lightning speed, namely those who had grown up with the terrycloth dummy. It was obvious that those who got to be with their own mother were the most secure. Perhaps it is not only softness and warmth that is needed to develop complete security?

PASSING DOWN TO THE NEXT GENERATION

Harlow's findings are in line with the results reported by Canadian researcher Michael Meaney from the McGill University. He demonstrated that some mother rats interact more than usual with their offspring by licking them, lying next to them and warming them during their first week of life. When these offspring became adult rats, they were less fearful, interacted more than other rats and were better able to handle stressful situations.

When these rats, in turn, became mothers, they were particularly caring and social towards their own offspring. This behaviour is then repeated in subsequent generations. Initially, it was believed that this behaviour was due to a genetic difference between rats that licked and interacted more and rats that interacted less. But Michael Meaney has carried out experiments where he has shown that this may not be the case. He showed that if the offspring born to a mother who devoted herself to them and interacted and licked a lot was taken from their real mother and instead raised by a mother who didn't lick or nurture them as much, the offspring adopted their 'foster-mother's' characteristics. They became more scared, less social and less stress resistant. Neither did they become more nurturing towards their own offspring when becoming mothers themselves. In the same way, it could also be shown that the offspring born to a mother who didn't lick as much, when raised by a more nurturing mother who licked a lot, adopted the 'foster-mother's' characteristics.

From these results, it was concluded that there was no real genetic difference between the rats that lick a lot and those that lick little. Instead, it was all about a character trait that was established in the first week of life and was dependent on how nurturing their mothers were and how much they licked their offspring during this time. The more licking and tactile interaction a rat pup was exposed to during the first week of life the more interactive and the calmer the rat became as an adult. It was the high amount of tactile stimulation that transformed them. Due to the fact that the closeness and the amount of licking also had an effect on the mothering behaviour of the mother rats and hence the next generation, it appeared to be a genetic difference. These apparent genetic differences have been shown to be due to the fact that the activity of certain genes can be influenced, i.e activated or deactivated, early in life. This phenomenon is called epigenetics.

CLOSENESS – A NEED IN ITSELF

Harlow's results from experiments with baby monkeys are fundamental in another way. What he reveals is that the babies not only like but are also drawn towards what is soft and warm. He performed an experiment where the babies got to choose between a steel wire dummy with a feeding bottle and a terrycloth dummy providing heat from a bulb but without the feeding bottle. It was shown that the babies basically spent all their time with the warm and woolly mother, although she had no food to give them. They were only with the steel wire dummy when they ate.

Harlow originally interpreted his findings as closeness being more important than nutrition. He eventually modified his interpretation to say that mother monkeys were also of great importance for the nutrient input to their offspring. Despite this small retreat, Harlow's research brought to attention something very important, namely that there is a distinct need for closeness which is separate from the need for nutrition. His experiments showed that the small baby monkeys looked for the warm and soft dummy even though 'she' had no food for them. They went to the steel wire dummy for food, but apart from that, they spent all their time with the terrycloth dummy, especially if they were afraid and needed to be consoled. The babies became calm and allowed themselves to be comforted, indicating that the closeness to the soft, warm terrycloth dummy actively exerted calming effects.

THE HUNGER OF SKIN

What Harlow didn't know, when he came to the conclusion that the closeness to the soft and warm terrycloth exerted an actively calming effect, was that sensory nerves originating in the skin are stimulated by heat and touch in order to create calm and social interaction. The author Ashley Montagu, in his book *Touching – The Human Significance of the Skin*, coined the term *skin hunger*, to describe the special need of closeness that was expressed in Harlow's experiments, a need which is satisfied by closeness, just like ordinary hunger (food hunger) is satisfied by food.

John Bowlby and attachment

Long before the concept of bonding was coined, the term attachment was used to describe the concept of something that united and kept humans together, but this phenomenon was believed to be created purely by mental processes and could, therefore, only be explained within the framework of psychological theory. However, the Englishman John Bowlby (1907–1990) changed this perspective. Bowlby, who was a physician, psychiatrist and psychoanalyst, was interested in the studies of imprinting behaviours carried out on animals by Lorenz. He began to see the child's attachment to its parents, and in particular to its mother, as a partly biological phenomenon. Bowlby suggested, just like Harlow, that a child seeks its mother to get closeness and love, and not just for food. From the positive experience of the mother (or another significant person) as a secure base to return to, the child begins to build its own self-esteem and security.

Bowlby considered attachment to be an innate necessary survival strategy – a way to ensure that the child received care and protection, in addition to closeness, love and security. He also said that the need for closeness to the mother of the slightly older child was activated only when the child became frightened or worried.

The importance of a child being with its parents was clearly illustrated when he wrote about the consequences of evacuation during the Second World War, when many children from London were sent to a temporary home in the countryside to avoid the dangers and horrors of the Blitz. In the aftermath, when examining the effects of evacuation on these children, it was found to everyone's surprise that those who had to leave their parents to live in the countryside were more psychologically unwell than those children who remained with their parents in bomb-shattered London.

John Bowlby interpreted these findings by suggesting that the children who experienced the terrors and horror during the Blitz were 'buffered against stressful experiences' because they had their parents with them. Those who were moved to other homes escaped the air-raids but were, instead, hit by the negative effects of being separated from their parents. When the children were separated from their parents, the soothing inner image of them faded and could not be maintained so worry increased.

Together with his colleague, Mary Ainsworth (1913–1999), John Bowlby has also described how a child's early relationship experiences can affect the development of an individual's future attachment style. For instance, studies of children who were cared for in hospitals over a long period of time showed the negative effect separations had on their attachment style and, later, their psychological well-being. Attachment to the mother was divided into three types: secure, insecure ambivalent and insecure avoidant. A secure attachment means broadly that the child can use his or her parent as a secure base to work from and a safe haven to return to when it becomes frightened, whereas a child with insecure attachment is, for a number of reasons, unable to use the parent to regulate its internal anxiety. The more responsive and accessible the primary caregivers are, the more secure the attachment style will be.

Ainsworth and Bowlby argued that our experiences of early relationships often affect how we as adults relate to others. We react in the same way as we did to our mothers or fathers in later relationships. However, Bowlby never ruled out that we can create positive attachments later in life regardless of the previous experiences that we carry around.

It should be emphasised that John Bowlby's contemporaries were not always so gracious in their judgement of his theories. During a lecture in England at which he was to describe his more biological approach to attachment theory rather than the prevailing psychoanalytical theories, everyone in the crowded lecture hall began booing and Bowlby was forced to leave the room.

CLOSENESS, TOUCH AND ATTACHMENT

Although Bowlby gave the phenomenon of attachment a more biological explanation than previous experts had done, he didn't link it to a physiological model of explanation. More modern techniques and methods have now made it possible to find out more about how humans look and function, which have in turn allowed us to explain why and how closeness is so important to our physical survival. But the fact is that John Bowlby's description of the child's attachment to the mother, and even Harry Harlow's findings, fit very well with the physiological model of closeness which is being introduced in this book and in which the active role of touch and closeness is emphasised.

3

How is the body controlled?

Most of what occurs in our body is controlled by the brain via the transmission of nerve signals that reach the different parts of the body and through hormones that reach their different target areas via the bloodstream. The arenas for these processes are the central nervous system, the peripheral nervous system, the hormone-producing glands and the hormones' target organs.

The central nervous system consists of two parts: the brain and the spinal cord. The peripheral nervous system, which can be divided into the voluntary and the involuntary or autonomic nervous system, consists of nerves that run outward and inward and that mediate contact between the body and the brain. In principle, both the central and peripheral nervous systems consist of nerves of different shapes and sizes. A neuron consists of a cell body with a number of projections. Those projections that receive impulses from other neurons are called dendrites and the ones that send impulses are known as axons.

As a rule, when a nerve cell is activated, neurotransmitters are released from the axon in order to reach receptors on another neuron or on the target organ. The neurotransmitters are, in fact, molecules that chemically mediate the signals from one nerve cell to another in the nervous system. These so-called neurotransmitters are stored in specialised swellings at the end of the axon. In response to a nerve impulse, the neurotransmitters are released into the synaptic junction which is the area in between the axon and the target cell.

Neurotransmitters, which mediate the activity between the two nerve cells, can consist of different chemicals. Some are amino acids, which are the building blocks of the proteins that the body produces, while others are peptides (amino acids linked together) and others are catecholamines (modified amino acids). Some gases can also serve as a messenger between the nerves as well as different types of fat molecules.

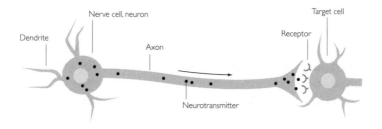

Schematic picture of a nerve cell (neuron).

The brain structure

The brain consists of several layers which from a developmental perspective have different ages. The brain can roughly be divided into the 'modern' cortex and the evolutionarily speaking older limbic system, the brainstem and the spinal cord. Farthest out is the convoluted cerebral cortex where various types of intellectual functions are processed and performed. These activities might involve strategic thinking, interpretation, evaluation and judgement.

Closest to the cerebral cortex is the limbic system. It is an important site for feelings, emotional impulses, memory and learning ability. The brainstem is the next layer and is located more deeply. The brainstem handles instincts, basic

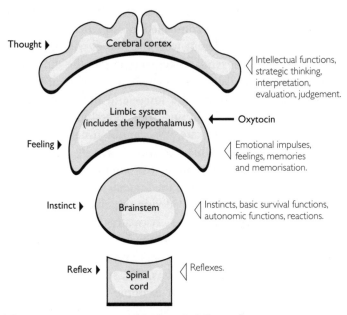

Schematic representation of the brain's different functions.

autonomic survival functions, and reactions. Finally, in the spinal cord, reflexes take place.

In both the older and newer parts of the brain, there are well defined areas associated with various types of activity. Knowledge of the brain's more specific and localised functions is growing rapidly mainly due to the fact that brain research over the last decades has had access to a number of techniques which in various ways have been able to highlight activity in the brain. Among the most common methods are CT scans (CAT scans), functional magnetic resonance imaging (fMRI) and positron emission tomography (PET scans).

Outgoing nerves or motor nerves

The movement of the muscles is controlled through the somatic nervous system. These nerves that emanate from the spinal cord have connections with the part of the cerebral cortex that control our body's movements. This means that the activity of these nerves is controlled by our will.

The situation is different with the nerves within the part of the peripheral nervous system known as the autonomic nervous system. These nerves regulate the activity of internal organs such as the heart, the lungs and the stomach, and thereby control our breathing, our digestion, our blood pressure and our heart rate. We cannot usually affect the functions of the autonomic nervous system by mind power alone. It is controlled, instead, by the older areas of the brain, such as the hypothalamus and the brainstem.

It is customary in turn to divide the autonomic nervous system into two parts: the sympathetic part and the parasympathetic part. To simplify the description of these two parts of the autonomic nervous system, you can say that they have different opposing functions. The sympathetic nervous system is linked to activity, for example in connection with movement or different stress reactions. The parasympathetic nervous system is related to rest and is responsible for the regulation of digestion and the storage of nutrients. These functions are mainly regulated by the vagal nerve, the nerve that connects many of the body's internal organs to the brain.

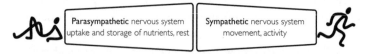

Schematic representation of the function of the parasympathetic and the sympathetic nervous system.

Incoming nerves or sensory nerves

The brain is constantly supplied with information from the outer and inner world. Through our senses, such as vision, hearing, smell and touch, we are informed about what is happening in the world around us and this information is then carried to the brain via our various sensory nerves.

The information from the world around us controls us more

than we are consciously aware of. Without us at first becoming aware of what is going on, thus without any information reaching the cerebral cortex, stimuli from the outside world can trigger fear and terror and fight-or-flight reactions. But our environment can also send us signals that all is calm and safe and then we respond with comfort, relaxation and calm. If sensory information comes via our skin or nose, these processes to a large extent take place unconsciously. However, even though this information is unconscious, it plays an important role in many ways in our relationships, which will be revealed in later chapters.

Hormones

In addition to the central nervous system, there is another important control and regulatory system: the endocrine or hormonal system. Hormones are molecules just like neurotransmitters, but they are released into the blood from the organ in which they are formed and the hormones reach their target organ via the blood. Most hormones are made in or released into the blood from a small organ in the brain called the pituitary gland, and are regulated by the hypothalamus, a region of the limbic system just above the pituitary gland. This area is of tremendous importance for the control and co-ordination of various bodily functions.

Another organ that produces lots of hormones is the gastrointestinal tract. The hormones in the gastrointestinal tract are also regulated by the hypothalamus but more indirectly via the vagal nerve. The hormones in the gastrointestinal tract, such as gastrin, cholecystokinin, and secretin, are important for proper digestion but also have important functions with regards to nutrient uptake, growth, appetite control and emotions. Gastrointestinal hormones reach different areas of the body via the bloodstream, but may also influence the brain through the activation of sensory nerves, e.g. the vagal nerve, from the digestive tract (see illustration on page 121).

The pituitary gland, where the majority of hormones are

made, consists of a frontal and dorsal lobe. The frontal pituitary lobe is responsible for the production of many important hormones, including those which control the production of milk, thyroid hormones, sex hormones and stress hormones.

Cortisol, which is also known as hydrocortisone, is a very important and vital hormone that keeps our blood pressure and blood sugar up. Without cortisol, you cannot live and this is why the blood always contains a certain level of this hormone. Large amounts of cortisol are secreted during stress and anxiety. A prolonged elevation of cortisol has several negative effects on the body. The most pronounced effects are that cortisol suppresses the immune system and significantly raises levels of glucose in the blood. (In contrast, during short-term elevated cortisol levels, the function of the immune system is enhanced.) In short, the regulation of cortisol, and also of ACTH or adrenocorticotropic hormone, the hormone released from the anterior pituitary and which controls cortisol secretion, is of vital importance for our health and well-being.

Cortisol production is regulated via the HPA axis (the hypothalamic-pituitary-adrenal axis). In the hypothalamus a control substance called CRF (corticotropin-releasing factor) is formed that is secreted to the frontal lobe of the pituitary gland via small blood vessels. CRF stimulates the release of the hormone ACTH (adrenocorticotropic hormone) which is produced in the frontal lobe of the pituitary gland and which, in turn, controls via the bloodstream the release of cortisol from the outer part of the adrenal gland, the adrenal cortex.

The hippocampus is the area of the brain which is connected to memory and learning ability and which is also an important switching station between different sensory impressions. Under normal circumstances, impulses from the hippocampus suppress the release of CRF in the hypothalamus and thus the activity of the whole HPA axis. If the hippocampal brake is released, the cortisol levels go through the roof. This can occur if the inhibitory effect normally exerted in the hippocampus by the cerebral cortex is blocked.

There are also CRF-containing nerves coming out from

the amygdala, which project to the locus coeruleus in the brainstem, an important regulatory centre for aggression, arousal and activation of the sympathetic nervous system. The amygdala is an important part of the limbic system, which is linked to the perception of fear. Cues from the outside are assessed in the amygdala as dangerous or not. If the surroundings are perceived as dangerous fear arises. In this way, elevated levels of CFR induce both mental and physical stress.

The HPA axis

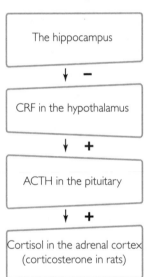

Illustration of the HPA axis that shows how the substance CRF, which is formed in the hypothalamus, controls the release of ACTH from the pituitary gland. ACTH reaches the adrenal gland through the bloodstream and stimulates release of cortisol from the adrenal cortex. CRF release in the hypothalamus is under inhibitory control via nerves from the hippocampus.

However, the dorsal lobe of the pituitary also releases hormones, namely oxytocin and vasopressin. Nerves containing these substances travel from the hypothalamus to the dorsal lobe of the pituitary gland, from which these substances are secreted into the bloodstream. In addition, oxytocin- and vasopressin-containing nerves also reach many other parts of the brain which they influence. In this way, the effects of oxytocin and vasopressin in the brain are co-ordinated with their hormonal effects.

How oxytocin works, and to some extent, vasopressin, will

be described in more detail in the next chapter, but here is a presentation of how oxytocin may influence our relationships, via the skin.

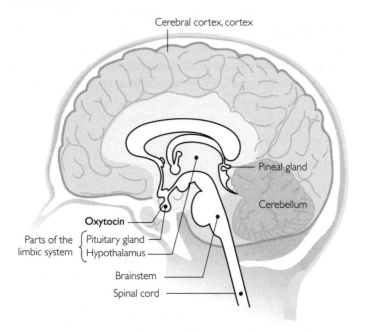

Illustration of a cross-section of the human brain showing the location of the hypothalamus and pituitary gland.

The skin – a pathway to oxytocin

In all of the various types of mammalian relationships mentioned in the first chapter, the substance oxytocin seems to play a key role for the relationship to become established and also to keep it established. This happens because oxytocin reduces fear of unknown individuals and also builds desire to be near and socially interact with others.

Oxytocin facilitates the recognition of 'other or others' by increasing the sensitivity of the different senses and the memorisation of these experiences. When the different individuals later interact, be it through closeness, sight, touch or smell, a sense of well-being and calm is created through oxytocin that connects and activates the signal systems that regulate these functions.

The signals that create oxytocin release reach the brain through our senses in the manner described above. It may be via odours, visual impressions or something that we hear. An often forgotten sensory organ is the skin, which is not only our oldest sensory organ but also our largest. In an adult, the surface of the skin is around 2m².

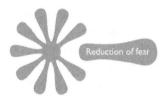

Reduction of fear

The characteristics of the skin

The skin develops from the ectoderm, the external layer of the three cell layers that form the embryo. Even the brain and the spinal cord derive from the ectoderm. The fact that the skin and the brain have a common developmental origin helps us understand why the skin isn't just a barrier to – but also an important link to – the world around us.

The author Ashley Montagu describes the relationship between the skin and the nervous system like this: 'Because the brain and the spinal cord develop as an indentation of the skin, it can be said that these two components of the nervous system consist of a part of the skin which is buried inside the body or that the skin is the part of the central nervous system which is exposed to the surroundings.'

The skin is the first of our senses that is developed. Already at the age of six weeks, an embryo responds to touch. Later on, the eyes and ears develop from the skin, as well as the senses of taste and smell. From a developmental viewpoint, the skin is a precursor to all our other senses, a kind of 'mother of the senses'. Because 'skin sense' is so ancient most of the information received by the skin is mediated through the older parts of the brain, where basic emotions and physiological reactions are regulated. Since the information we receive from the skin is not very clear and conscious and since the reactions caused by such stimuli can't be influenced by will, we tend to underestimate the information from the skin. Instead, we overemphasise the importance of our impressions from considerably more 'modern' sense organs such as our ears and, in particular, our eyes.

This oversight of the skin's ability to receive information from the world around us and convey it to the brain is most probably the reason why, within medicine, the skin's intermediary role in connection with closeness and relationships has been underestimated, and instead explanatory models of a purely psychological nature have been created.

Sensory receptors and sensory nerves

In the skin, there are a number of small structures or sensory receptors that react to different types of information from the world around us. They can be activated by injury, poisonous substances or temperature differences but also through pressure or touch.

The information obtained by the sensory receptors of the skin, as a response to different environmental stimuli, is then transmitted to the sensory nerves. Through these sensory nerves, this information reaches the spinal cord from the rear and there they connect to other nerves, which travel upwards in the spinal cord to reach the brain. The skin is obviously in very close connection with the brain and other parts of the nervous system.

The sensory nerves convey information to the brain about a variety of different conditions in the skin, including pain, touch, temperature (heat and cold) and various degrees of pressure. It is customary to divide the nerves from the skin into thin and thick nerve fibres.

The thick nerve fibres are surrounded by a layer of fat (the myelin layer). These nerves are quick firing and give rise to acute signals when the skin is touched or damaged. In particular, the experience of touch is transmitted via the coarser nerve fibres.

The thinner, so-called C-fibres transmit nerve impulses more slowly and are, from a developmental standpoint, older than the thicker ones. They don't give rise to a clear, localised sensation and have previously been considered to be connected to more diffuse experiences of pain. Toothache is a typical example, where, even with very severe pain, it can be difficult to specify exactly which tooth it is that hurts.

Gothenburg researchers, Åke Vallbo and Håkan Olausson, have recently discovered that a part of the C-fibres, the so called CT-fibres, also respond to touch. However, they don't respond to just any kind of touch but react especially to soft and caressing strokes across the skin at a rate of one centimetre per second. These strokes have also been shown to activate a part of the brain called the insula that is connected to the experiences of well-being.

Håkan Olausson and his colleagues have examined a Canadian family that lacks the usual thick myelinated sensory nerves, but still have the thinner type of sensory nerves. With the aid of fMRI, a technique that makes areas in the brain that are being activated during certain processes light up stronger than its surroundings, it was shown that the insula is still activated by touch in members of the family, but only through stroking of the skin at a rate of one centimetre per second. This finding supports the assumption that the CT-fibres have an important function in the way touch is perceived.

There is yet another type of thin sensory nerve of the C-fibre type that sends information from the skin to the brain. These nerve fibres bypass the spinal cord and reach the brain together with the vagal nerve, the nerve that connects many of the body's internal organs to the brain. These nerves extend mainly from the skin on the chest and the front of the body and from the uterus and the vagina. They have a very direct contact with the hypothalamus and the oxytocin-producing cells, and therefore they have an important function when it comes to regulating different mental and bodily functions.

Defence or peace and quiet via the skin

If the skin is exposed to any form of stimulation which is dangerous to the organism, different types of deterrence and defensive reactions (fight-or-flight response) are triggered via the sympathetic nervous system, and in addition the HPA axis is activated. If the skin, instead, perceives the surroundings as innocuous or perhaps even pleasant and positive, different types of reaction patterns are triggered which are associated with peace and quiet. In this context, the defence and stress reactions are suppressed and processes linked to the parasympathetic nervous system related to growth and healing are strengthened.

When the sensory nerves are activated, a composite effect pattern is created because effects are triggered at different levels during the nerve impulses' journey from the skin to the brain. Effects are generated both before and after the nerve impulses have reached the brain, and both the older and the newer parts of the brain are influenced. It is via the effects in the sensory cortex that we become aware of where and when we've been touched or injured. In the older parts of the brain, the nerve impulses can affect our mood, create pain or pleasure and influence bodily functions, such as stress levels, blood pressure and digestion. To illustrate this, we will follow a pain nerve and a touch nerve on its way from the skin to the brain.

How do the pain nerves work?

The individual who becomes the victim of some kind of unpleasant or painful type of contact typically reacts by trying to avoid the danger. Through effects in the sensory cortex, you become aware when a painful stimulus is affecting the skin. But you also pull away the hand which has been damaged or burned and you also run away from the person who slaps you or perhaps give a slap back if you dare. The latter effects could be of a reflexive nature and could, therefore, be triggered within the spinal cord.

But the pain nerves work on several levels. Locally, around a wound or where any poison has ended up on the skin, an inflammatory reaction is triggered in the skin to drive out or destroy the harmful material. These local reactions are partly due to the pain nerves having small arms or extensions that run backwards to the site of origin of the sensory nerve in the skin. These extensions contain substances that may cause inflammation when they are released into the surrounding tissues.

When a pain nerve is stimulated, nerve impulses travel to the spinal cord and from there on to the brain to influence behaviour and to induce stress reactions such as an increased activity in the sympathetic nervous system and in the HPA axis, as will be described below. At the same time the tiny nerve branches that run backwards (the axon reflexes) are activated and the substances that may create local inflammatory reactions in the skin are secreted from the extensions. In addition, the pain nerves can affect and give rise to reflexive movements when they reach the spinal cord.

When the nerve impulses finally reach the cerebral cortex a conscious feeling of pain is created, as described above. But the pain-conducting nerves may also cause diffuse pain and inflammation via effects in the more original and older parts of the brain. These effects can occur with a slight delay. Once the pain signals reach the hypothalamus the body's stress system is also triggered. The HPA axis is activated and the heart rate and blood pressure may rise due to an activation of the sympathetic nervous system. In principle, the individual defends himself on all levels and all these effects are consequences of the activation of pain-mediating nerve fibres.

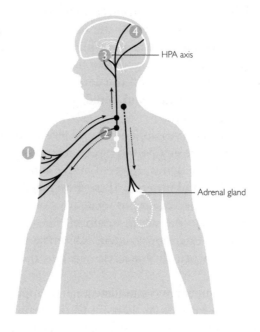

When pain nerves are activated, effects are created on many different levels in the nervous system. Small nerve branches, the so called axon reflexes, depart from the pain-mediating sensory nerves to go 'backwards' toward the skin (1). In the spinal cord, nerve fibres that project back to the site from where the pain impulse originated may be activated, the so-called spinal reflexes (2). Effects can also take place in the older parts of the brain, including the hypothalamus (3) and, of course in the cerebral cortex (4) where the experience of the nerve impulses becomes conscious. Note that in the hypothalamus painful stimuli cause a stress reaction, which involves the HPA axis being activated and the release of cortisol from the adrenal gland.

How do the touch nerves function?

When something or someone touches us, we almost immediately experience the sense of being touched and where on the body it's occurring. These are experiences that are created in the sensory cortex – the area of the cerebral cortex where tactile information is handled. But this is not the only thing that happens because the 'touch nerves', both the thin and the thick ones, are active on several other levels in the spinal cord and the brain.

The incoming touch nerves have small branches already in the skin, which go backwards. When a touch nerve is activated, impulses are simultaneously triggered in the main part of the sensory nerve that projects to the spinal cord and in the small branches that travel backwards to the skin. The latter results in an increased blood flow in the area that was touched, since substances that dilate blood vessels are released from the small backward-running fibres. In this way the skin becomes a bit warmer, which may be perceived as a pleasant sensation. When the nerve impulses reach the spinal cord, new reflexes are activated. Some of them return to the area that was touched (spinal reflex arc), which contributes to the feeling of warmth and well-being. Furthermore, touch can reduce pain by inhibiting the activity in ingoing 'pain nerves' when they enter the spinal cord.

Prior to reaching the sensory cortex in the modern part of the brain, the nerves that transmit the touch impulses branch off to the older part of the brain, including areas in the brainstem and in the hypothalamus where important basic functions are regulated. Touch stimulates the release of oxytocin into the brain, which means that among other things stress responses are subdued. Some of these effects, but not all, occur with a slight delay in comparison with the perception that the body is being touched, since they are exerted in the much older part of the brain. The effects of touch are created at several levels and in several steps in the same manner as harmful and painful stimuli trigger effects at multiple levels in the nervous system.

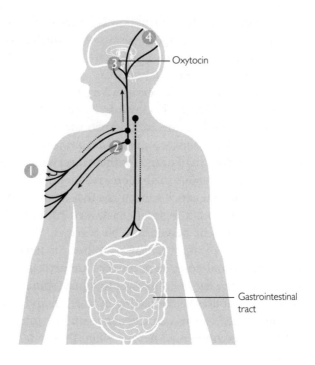

Touch induces effects at the same levels and via similar mechanisms in the brain as does pain. But the nerve signals that are created by touch lead to the release of oxytocin, thereby triggering oxytocin-mediated effects, such as the activation of the gastrointestinal tract.

Now you have a basic idea of how the body's nervous and endocrine systems work, both of which have a bearing on how we feel and experience ourselves in the world around us. A large part of this world consists of close and less close relationships. Since oxytocin released through touch plays an important role in these relationships, it is the focus of this book. So, let's move on to oxytocin!

4

What is oxytocin?

Earlier in this book, we discussed oxytocin and looked at where it is formed and how it is transported in the body. As previously mentioned, oxytocin is a substance which is released into the circulation from the pituitary dorsal lobe. It was originally associated with childbirth and lactation, but is now also known to be related to touch, closeness and nutrition. This chapter will describe in detail what is known today about the many effects of oxytocin, especially in the context of relationships.

The discovery of oxytocin

In 1909, the Englishman Sir Henry Dale discovered that an extract from the pituitary dorsal lobe caused contractions of the uterus in pregnant cats. He gave the substance the name oxytocin, which means 'quick birth' in Greek. A few years later he discovered that oxytocin also stimulated the contractions of the alveoli, small containers which store the milk in the mammary gland. Through these contractions, the ejection of milk is triggered.

Soon after the discovery of the effects of oxytocin by Dale, the substance started to be used to induce and accelerate contractions in women during labour. The reason for this was that the chemical structure of oxytocin and its effects on the uterine muscles are identical in all mammals.

What is not as well known is that oxytocin also co-ordinates a whole array of adaptations with regards to behaviour and bodily functions which are connected to birthing and lactation. This happens because oxytocin is linked to other well known signalling systems in the brain. In fact, oxytocin works in the same way as an important co-ordinating factor in other types of mammalian relationships, and this applies both to pair and group relationships. Oxytocin exerts its effects in the context of relationships in a unique way by connecting and triggering effects which are mediated via other signalling systems.

Protein and signalling substance

Oxytocin is evolutionarily speaking a very old substance, a small protein that is chemically identical in all mammals. Oxytocin is mainly formed in two large groups of nerve cells in the brain called the supraoptic and paraventricular nuclei. They are both located in the hypothalamus, an ancient part of the brain – a sort of 'control station' that exists in all mammals and more primitive animals. Basic functions, such as the pulse and blood pressure, hunger and thirst, aggression and sexuality, are regulated by the hypothalamus. The release of most of our hormones is also controlled from here.

The many effects of oxytocin

In addition to the effects found in childbirth and lactation, it has been shown that oxytocin plays an important role in many other contexts. This is partly due to the fact that the oxytocin that is formed in the nerves of the hypothalamus can act via several different pathways.

Three possible paths

The oxytocin nerves reach the pituitary posterior lobe and are transported into the bloodstream where oxytocin serves as a hormone. These nerve fibres have their origin in a specific type of oxytocin-producing cell, the magnocellular neurons (the big cells) originating from the supraoptic or the parvocellular nucleus. Other oxytocin nerves reach important regulatory regions in the brain, and oxytocin then acts as a neurotransmitter. These nerves may have their origin in magnocellular neurons or parvocellular neurons (small neurons) originating from the paraventricular nucleus. In other words, oxytocin acts partly as a hormone via the bloodstream and partly as a neurotransmitter via oxytocin-producing nerve cells in the brain. It might also be able to 'leak' via diffusion, directly from the nerve cells, to different surrounding parts of the brain. One of the reasons why oxytocin has such a broad effect spectrum is because it may act through these three different mechanisms.

VIA THE BLOOD

The oxytocin which is produced in the magnocellular neuron in the hypothalamus is sent down to the pituitary posterior lobe via the oxytocin-producing nerve's long axons. Oxytocin is released from the axons in the posterior pituitary into a network of small blood vessels and from there on it passes into the blood circulation. The oxytocin in the blood then affects, for example, the uterine contractions during labour and the expulsion of milk during lactation. When oxytocin exerts effects via the bloodstream, they are called endocrine or hormonal effects.

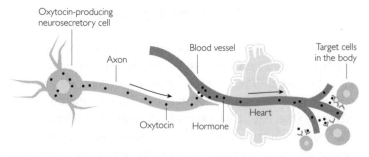

Oxytocin as a hormone affects receptors of the target cells via transportation in the bloodstream.

VIA THE NERVES

Some of the oxytocin-producing nerves emanating from the parvocellular neurons in the paraventricular nucleus of the hypothalamus don't project to the posterior pituitary lobe, but instead reach many other important regulatory areas of the brain, thereby forming a network of nerve fibres through which oxytocin can produce co-ordinated patterns of effects. When oxytocin is released from the nerve endings of the oxytocin-producing nerve cells in the brain, it works as a neurotransmitter.

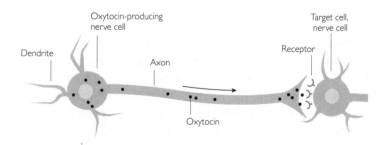

Oxytocin as a neurotransmitter affects receptors located on other nerve cells.

VIA DIFFUSION

In addition, large amounts of oxytocin are released directly from oxytocin-producing nerve cell bodies and their dendrites, the shorter and incoming projections on the oxytocin-producing cells in the supraoptic and paraventricular nuclei. As oxytocin diffuses into the surrounding tissue the levels of oxytocin may become very high and therefore oxytocin may affect the function of other types of nerve cells without these cells being reached by the oxytocin nerves. Oxytocin can probably also be transported quite far away from the oxytocin-producing cells in the brain and can therefore also affect more distant parts of the brain. When oxytocin exerts effects in this way, it is said that it exerts paracrine effects.

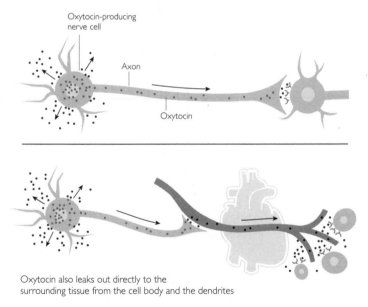

Oxytocin also leaks out directly to the surrounding tissue from the cell body and the dendrites

Oxytocin-producing cells, whether they connect to another nerve cell in the brain or send oxytocin into the bloodstream, can when being intensely stimulated also send out oxytocin via the nerve cell body and the small incoming 'dendrites'. Oxytocin could then reach the surrounding tissues via diffusion.

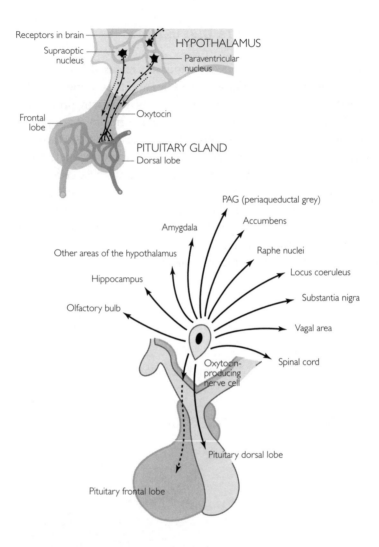

Top illustration: *Oxytocin nerves from the hypothalamus project to the posterior lobe of the pituitary gland where oxytocin is released into the blood. Oxytocinergic nerves also project to other areas of the brain, where oxytocin affects different functions in the brain via oxytocin receptors located on other nerve cells.*

Lower illustration: *Oxytocin is transported to the pituitary dorsal lobe (and is brought out into the blood for hormonal effects), the pituitary frontal lobe (stimulates the release of growth hormone and prolactin and reduces the release of ACTH), the olfactory bulb (affects the sense of smell), the hippocampus (centre for memory and learning, and regulation of the HPA axis), the amygdala (regulation of fear and social interaction), the PAG (centre for the regulation of pain and inflammation), other areas in the hypothalamus (centre for stress, appetite and fluid regulation), the raphe nuclei (centre for the production of serotonin, relevant to mood states), the locus coeruleus (centre for norepinephrine production, which is of importance for levels of alertness and aggression), the substantia nigra and nucleus accumbens (centres for dopamine production, which is of importance for concentration and movement as well as reward), the vagal area (centre for the in- and outgoing parasympathetic vagal nerve fibres and for the function of the sympathetic nervous system) and the spinal cord (in particular the area involved in pain transmission and the sympathetic nerve system's in- and-outgoing nerve fibres).*

Oxytocin receptors

When oxytocin has been transported to its target organs, it must bind to a receiver, a receptor, in order to exert its effects. The structure of the receptor that affects the contractions of the uterus has long been known. This type of receptor is also available in many other places, both in the brain and in the rest of the body. However, there are oxytocin receptors with different kinds of properties, including one that conveys the calming and relaxing effects and perhaps another one that creates the refreshing effects. The function of some oxytocin receptors is increased by the female hormone oestrogen and, in this way, some of the effects of oxytocin can be enhanced by oestrogen and consequently more strongly expressed in women.

The effects of oxytocin

Oxytocin is released via nerves in the brain and can lead to a variety of effects that might be expressed in the context of relationships. In principle, social interactions are stimulated, stress levels are reduced and healing processes stimulated. These effects will be described in more detail in later chapters.

The HPA axis

In order to understand how oxytocin works we might need to look in more detail at the way in which oxytocin reduces the activity in the HPA axis since it illustrates how oxytocin works on a wide front. If, for example, oxytocin is given to rats, there is a reduction in the levels of corticosterone, which corresponds to the human stress hormone cortisol. Oxytocin reduces the cortisol concentration in several ways based on the principle that 'every little helps'. It is by acting at many different levels and by co-ordinating these effects that oxytocin becomes so powerful.

The HPA axis

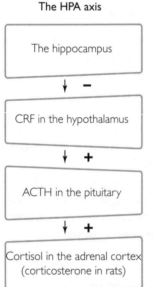

Oxytocin can decrease the activity in the HPA axis, and hence the secretion of cortisol, by influencing the function of all the different steps in the HPA axis. The inhibition of CRF release from the hippocampus is amplified, amd in addition CRF, ACTH and cortisol release are counteracted by oxytocin in the hypothalamus, in the pituitary and in the adrenal cortex respectively.

Autonomic nervous system

Oxytocin also affects the activity in the autonomic nervous system which, as we have seen, consists of the sympathetic part (primarily connected to movement and activity) and the parasympathetic part (primarily connected to nutritional storage, growth and repair).

Oxytocin lowers blood pressure by suppressing the activity of the sympathetic nervous system and lowers the pulse rate by increasing the activity in the parasympathetic nervous system. Both of these effects are due to oxytocin being released from nerves projecting from the hypothalamus to areas of the brainstem that are important for regulation of the activity of the autonomic nervous system, where the two 'pair-horses' – the sympathetic and the parasympathetic nervous systems – belong. It is partly by increasing the activity in the parasympathetic nervous system and through corresponding mechanisms in the brain that oxytocin stimulates growth and healing.

Other signalling systems

Another reason why oxytocin has such a broad spectrum of effects is that it not only acts by activating its own receptors but also triggers other well-known signalling systems, for example dopamine (regulation of movement and reward), serotonin (involved in the regulation of mood and satiation) and acetylcholine (involved in memory and learning processes and regulation of activity in the gastrointestinal tract). Oxytocin exerts its analgesic effects by influencing the function of endogenous opiates (endorphins and enkephalins) and several of its anti-stress effects are exerted by blocking the activity in the brain's noradrenergic signalling system.

Oxytocin has the ability to connect the effects from different signalling systems into patterns and consequently the hormone can produce combinations of effects which are expressed in connection with different types of relationships.

Oxytocin release is at the same time affected by the activity in other signalling systems. Most neurotransmitters stimulate oxytocin release but, in contrast, the endogenous opiates have the effect of blocking oxytocin release. In this way, chains of effects are formed.

Short- and long-term effects

When oxytocin is administered on a single occasion, blood pressure and stress levels are reduced for a few hours. Oxytocin only 'survives' for a few minutes in the bloodstream and for approximately half an hour in the brain. But if oxytocin is given several times, the effects can persist for weeks. How can this be?

This is because oxytocin activates other signalling systems in the short term and alters their functions on a more long-term basis. In this way, oxytocin becomes an effective 'hider'. It disappears quickly but the effects remain. This happens because:

- More neurotransmitters may be produced
- The receptor's ability to bind the neurotransmitters may increase
- The number of receptors may increase

Opposing effects

Oddly enough, oxytocin can also have the opposite stress-like effect, that is, it may temporarily increase the heart rate, the blood pressure and cortisol levels. As described above, oxytocin is not always the last link in the effect chain but is more of a co-ordinator of the effect patterns that are expressed in different situations and is, therefore, partly dependent on the situation itself. Various forms of closeness can lead to a reduction in blood pressure by stimulating the release of oxytocin in the brain.

In contrast, during birth oxytocin creates an increase in blood pressure via hormonal effects to ensure that the mother and the offspring or baby get enough oxygenated blood and nutrients. The inner and outer environment influences the way that the effects of oxytocin are expressed. It appears that the calming and stress-relieving effects come to a peak expression in a familiar, quiet and secure environment. In an unfamiliar and frightening environment, or when stress levels are high as during labour, oxytocin can produce the opposite effect.

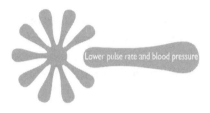

Lower pulse rate and blood pressure

Oxytocin fragments

The truth is that the oxytocin molecule can be divided into different 'parts' which are linked to different effects. An oxytocin molecule (which is a peptide or small protein) consists of nine amino acids that are connected in a certain way. Normally, six amino acids form a circle and from this circle 'a small tail' made from three amino acids sticks out. It is primarily this form of oxytocin that is circulating as a hormone in the bloodstream. It is needed for the stimulation of contractions of the uterine muscles during labour and the expulsion of milk during lactation.

In the brain, the circle is often opened up and, instead, a new type of oxytocin is formed that consists of eight amino acids in a row and a branch consisting of only one amino acid. This variant of oxytocin is calming. This long molecule can be broken down into even smaller parts or fragments that are stimulating or calming.

Some of oxytocin's functions – the contraction of muscles in the uterus and the mammary glands, and social interaction versus calm and relaxation (anti-stress) and growth – seem to belong together and to be linked to separate parts of the mother oxytocin molecule. These oxytocin fragments do not appear to bind to the same receptors. There are also probably several other oxytocin fragments which exert specific effects and which perhaps bind to until now uncharacterised oxytocin receptors.

Vasopressin, the sibling of oxytocin

If you exchange two of the amino acids in oxytocin, you get a molecule called vasopressin. Vasopressin is also formed in the hypothalamus and can, just like oxytocin, be both a hormone and a neurotransmitter in the brain. The three main tasks of vasopressin are:

- Reducing the production of urine. (A slightly changed vasopressin molecule, DAVP, may be given as a medicine to children who wet the bed. Since DAVP suppresses the production of urine, it is easier for the child to stay dry at night.)
- To raise blood pressure by contracting the muscles around the blood vessels.
- To influence behaviour. (Animal studies have shown that the administration of vasopressin causes aggressiveness. The animals that received vasopressin created larger territories and became more attacking. The bonding connection between individuals, particularly in males, was also affected.)

An age-old pair

Oxytocin and vasopressin are opposites. Oxytocin creates positive social interactions, and a feeling of calm and relaxation and lowering of blood pressure. In contrast, vasopressin creates aggressive interactions and raises the level of stress, which manifests itself in increased blood pressure. Both substances co-ordinate the behaviour and bodily functions into patterns which are appropriate in certain situations. But there are, of course, also other 'control substances' which have a co-ordinating function.

Oxytocin

Tyr   Cys

Ile   Cys — Pro — Leu — Gly   (NH₂)

Glu   Asn

Vasopressin

Tyr   Cys

Phe   Cys — Pro — Arg — Gly   (NH₂)

Glu   Asn

Illustration of the chemical structure of oxytocin and vasopressin.
The 'balls' represent individual amino acids. Both substances contain
nine amino acids of which seven are in common. It is through the two
different amino acids that the different effect patterns are created.

The effect of oxytocin in humans

The oxytocin that is released in the brain during childbirth and lactation increases the mother's capacity for social interaction, induces a sense of calmness and makes her feel good. She becomes less stressed, more relaxed and more nutrient-efficient. This is what the next chapter will be about.

Scientific reports are now starting to appear that show that men who have been given oxytocin react in the same way. In these studies oxytocin has been given by nasal spray. This works because only a very thin skeletal wall separates the nose from the brain and since the blood brain barrier that normally hinders circulating substances like oxytocin from entering the brain is very weak in this area. Oxytocin given as nasal spray can, therefore, easily pass into the circulation of the brain via the small blood vessels in the nasal wall.

The Swiss researcher, Marcus Heinrichs has studied what happens when oxytocin spray is given to men. The men who receive oxytocin become less fearful. This effect has, for example, been shown by letting the men watch unpleasant pictures while studying their brains with fMRI scans. The activity in the amygdala – the area of the brain that is activated during anxiety and danger – was measured. Typically, it can be seen that activity increases in the amygdala when a participant sees a threatening face. Among the men that received oxytocin spray, the activation of the amygdala was not as strong as in the control group who received saline spray (placebo) instead. The oxytocin spray also reduced the fear experienced in the men who watched an unpleasant and frightening film and their levels of the stress hormone, cortisol, decreased.

The oxytocin-treated men's ability to deal with social interactions was also amplified. They looked more into the eyes of others and they were, for example, able to decide with greater certainty the emotional state of individuals depicted. It has been shown that oxytocin activates several of the areas of the brain related to social interactions. Finally, it was found that the men who were treated with oxytocin became more trusting and generous.

In summary

- Oxytocin is a small substance that is formed in nerve cells in the hypothalamus in the brain.
- Some oxytocin nerves go down into the pituitary dorsal lobe and, from there, oxytocin enters the bloodstream and goes further into the body.
- Oxytocin nerves also reach other areas of the brain, including centres involved in regulation of fear and social relationships.
- In addition, oxytocin nerves go to the areas of the brain that affect the degree of well-being, calm, pain sensitivity, the levels of stress hormones and heart rate,

blood pressure and the activity in the gastrointestinal tract.

- Oxytocin is released in connection with different types of relationships and contributes to the enabling and the initiation of the relationship and makes it more permanent, partly by speeding up the recognition and the memory of the other person and partly through the connection of positive experiences to the closeness or the presence of the other person or persons.
- This is possible because the oxytocin nerves reach so many areas in the brain and can create different combinations of effects.
- The effects of the administration of oxytocin spray in men are being studied. It has been found that the effects produced are consistent to those induced when oxytocin has been administered to rats. This shows that the oxytocin effects are part of our mammalian inheritance, which also means that they will not necessarily become conscious and that we cannot influence them through our will.

5

Oxytocin and attachment

The second chapter described attachment theory and bonding and its relation to the closeness model, which runs like a red thread through this book. The role of oxytocin in relation to the development of bonding and attachment will be described more fully in this chapter.

At the beginning of life

When a new baby is born into this world it's a kind of miracle. And yet, it is something that has been repeated in the same way in countless generations. Although every birth is unique, the way that women give birth has not changed (unless interfered with). And across the world, mothers and their babies interact in the same way, when the baby is born. Many parents will be truly fascinated that their newborn can do so many things. When, for example, the baby is placed on the mother's tummy, it moves towards her breast, starts to suckle and seeks eye contact. The mother also knows how to welcome the baby. How come this is the case? Well, the fact is that these behaviours are innate and part of our ancient instincts which manifest themselves when a child is born.

The newborn child feels good when it is very close to its

parents and the mother (or father) feels good as well. The closeness increases the contact between the two and makes them feel more content and calmer. This early interaction affects the parents and the child straight after the birth and probably also for life, because it lays a special foundation for the ability to trust, for social interaction and the sense of calm and quiet.

Many mammals show similar patterns associated with birthing. The instinctive behaviour that the parents and children express during birth is the part of the 'mammalian heritage' that was described in the first chapter. The reason why these instincts have survived to this day is because they have had, and still have, a great survival value.

Oxytocin increases maternal behaviour

In a number of studies of mammals, it has been shown that the mother's nurturing of her offspring is stimulated if oxytocin is supplied to the brain. If, for example, female rats receive oxytocin, their interaction increases both with their own offspring and indeed also with the offspring of other rats (they therefore need not have given birth to them themselves); they build nests, lick, feed and defend the offspring more actively than if they hadn't been given oxytocin. The maternal behaviour is expressed in different ways in different species, but even cows, ewes and female apes increase their care for their offspring if they receive extra oxytocin and it also accelerates the attachment process.

Normally, maternal behaviour is stimulated by the oxytocin that is released during birth and in relation to lactation. However, if the effect of oxytocin is blocked in the new mammal mother, their nurturing behaviour is absent. This has been demonstrated in sheep and cows with the aid of an oxytocin antagonist or with the aid of epidural anaesthesia, which blocks the nerves that are involved in oxytocin release during labour. The direct bonding process is absent here too. But if oxytocin is administered, the maternal behaviour returns.

The effects of oxytocin in the mother-child relationship

Oxytocin plays a key role in the relationship between the animal mother and its offspring by activating and co-ordinating in an ingenious way different effects that are of importance for the two of them from both a short- and a long-term perspective. Despite the many differences between the mammalian species, there are fundamental similarities concerning oxytocin's contribution with regards to maternal behaviour.

Oxytocin facilitates the contact between the mother and the offspring as the fear of unknown individuals is suspended, while at the same time, social interaction is stimulated. These effects take place, for example, in the part of the brain called the amygdala. Oxytocin enhances the sense of smell and allows the mother and offspring to more rapidly recognise each other's scent. In this way, by facilitating learning and the memory of the scent, they quickly learn to recognise each other.

Recognition and attachment

Taking care of the offspring is facilitated by oxytocin's ability to connect different movements and behaviours to create a behavioural 'nursing program'. For example, by switching on the body's reward system – in particular endogenous opioids and dopamine in an area of the brain called the nucleus accumbens – and by creating calm and relaxation (subdued activity in the stress axis and the sympathetic nervous system) the closeness becomes pleasant. This contributes towards keeping mother and offspring together, because these effects subside when they are no longer close to each other.

Oxytocin is released through nutrition and closeness

The offspring are also affected by oxytocin, partly through the actual suckling during lactation and partly because the milk that they drink leads to the release of certain hormones from the gastrointestinal tract, such as cholecystokinin (CCK). When CCK is released in the small intestine, the ascending nerve fibres of the vagal nerve, which connect the gastrointestinal tract with the brain, are activated. This in turn leads to a release of oxytocin into the brain. The milk is calming, especially if it is fatty and contains proteins, and this speeds up the attachment to the mother. But the act of suckling in itself, the touch and closeness to the animal mother all contribute – through oxytocin, a substance which is found in all mammals – to create well-being, reduce anxiety, stimulate social interaction, stimulate growth, and speed up the attachment between offspring and mother.

Pregnancy and childbirth

Most parents already have a close relationship with their child during pregnancy, even if they've just felt it kick and seen the outlines of it on the ultrasound screen. And the mother is affected both physically and mentally throughout pregnancy by the pregnancy hormones oestrogen and progesterone in order to be able to welcome the expectant child. But the first real meeting takes place only when the baby is born.

The role of oxytocin

During childbirth, the amount of oxytocin in the blood increases greatly in the woman, and this triggers the contractions so that the baby can be born. Oxytocin is released in short pulses that progressively become more frequent. Towards the end of labour, there are only a few minutes between the contractions. When the baby's head pushes on the cervix, sensory nerves are stimulated and they send information to the oxytocin-producing areas in the hypothalamus via the spinal cord. The more the baby is pushing, the more oxytocin is released and the greater the contractions of the uterus. Oxytocin also activates and co-ordinates certain effects into a particular pattern which is appropriate during birth. Because of this, the oxytocin nerves in the brain that reduce pain are also activated. Oxytocin also helps to raise blood pressure during labour (via circulating effects) so that the mother, and the baby via the placenta, get enough nutrition and oxygen during the contractions.

The mother is prepared to meet the child

Human mothers are also psychologically affected by the birth, but in a more subtle way than other mammals. Studies carried out on new mothers show that they are often calmer and more interested in social interactions compared to women of the same age who haven't given birth. Two days after the birth, most mothers have become so profoundly adjusted to care for their children that in psychological tests and self-assessment questionnaires they describe themselves as less anxious, less aggressive and more socially interested and competent than they have been in the past. They also no longer have the same need for variation but prefer a more mundane life. This adjustment of the mother's psyche is a part of the human mini-version of the maternal behaviour that is triggered by childbirth or administration of oxytocin in sheep and other mammals.

Caesarean section and epidural

In mothers who give birth by Caesarean section or in those who receive an epidural in labour (a local anaesthetic of some parts of the spinal cord to reduce the pain of childbirth), the development of these mental adaptations which are mediated via oxytocin is delayed. Mothers who give birth by Caesarean section have either had a relatively short period of labour, or perhaps no labour at all, and hence no or a very much reduced oxytocin release. An epidural anaesthetic not only blocks the activity in the nerves in the spinal cord that transmit pain, but also in the nerves that lead to the release of oxytocin normally triggered when the baby's head is pushing against the cervix. Consequently, mothers who receive an epidural also have lower levels of oxytocin during labour.

It is only after a period of lactation that these mothers develop the oxytocin-dependent maternal adaptations. As each individual breastfeed leads to a release of oxytocin, the repetition of feeds ultimately creates a similar adjustment like the strong oxytocin release that occurs in childbirth.

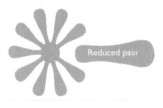

The first meeting

After the birth, if all has gone well, the mother is prepared for the first meeting with her baby. The oxytocin that has been released affects her brain so that she will be less scared and more calm. She becomes more interested in her child and more responsive to its signals. Her ability to experience positive emotions is heightened as is the ability to bond with the newborn baby.

In Sweden, it is now routine to put the newborn baby on the mother's (or father's) chest after the birth to help the parents and the child to bond as soon as possible and for the experience of the first meeting to be as positive as possible. It is a return to a more primitive and natural approach. It was only when childbirth was moved from the home to the hospital that it became routine to separate the mother and child after the birth, a procedure that obviously did not occur during home births.

If you observe what happens when the baby is placed on the mother's tummy, you can see that the two act and interact with each other according to some kind of pattern. The baby, which at first is calm and still, gradually begins to move its hands, both towards its mouth and towards the mother's breast. It then starts to crawl towards the breast and often manages to start suckling all by itself. The baby is now very alert and awake and looking for eye contact with its mother. However, after around one or two hours, the baby becomes tired and falls asleep, whether it's been able to suckle or not.

Meanwhile, the mother examines her baby using sight and touch, and starts talking to it. Often she feels calm and very proud and happy. She is filled with love for the irresistible, cute baby that she thinks is the most beautiful baby in the world. She wants to hold the baby, feed it and help it in every possible way.

The temperature rises

Beyond what we can see with our eyes there are also other types of communication going on between the mother and the child. When she sees and feels her baby, the temperature of her chest rises and starts to pulse. The rapid temperature increase is probably due to blood vessels in the skin of the chest dilating or widening so that she can warm her child. The child reacts to the mother's warmth by relaxing. As a result the blood vessels in the skin of the child also dilate and its skin temperature increases, and the warmer the mother is, the higher the temperature of the child. This is most noticeable on the child's feet, which turn pink. To provide warmth is a more universal skill than giving milk, and fathers can of course also give warmth if they have skin-to-skin contact with their newborn after the birth. The ability to provide warmth from the chest is reminiscent of the bird mother, who picks her feathers from her chest and dilates her blood vessels so that she can warm the eggs that she is brooding.

The closeness to the mother or the father also makes the baby feel calm and safe and it cries less than if it was lying in its own bed next to them. There is an association between the pink feet and the calmness. A person who is calm has warm feet because the blood circulation to the feet is open. If, on the other hand, a person is worried, the blood vessels contract and the feet become cold. It is this correlation that is described when we say that someone gets cold feet or, in other words, has become afraid.

Pheromones

In parallel with the communication taking place via the temperature, there is also a mutual influence via pheromones, which among other things accelerate the development of bonding and attachment between the mother/father and child. Pheromones are also found in insects, fish and other mammals. In humans they are formed in sweat, urine, breastmilk and in the skin on the hands and feet. Pheromones are tiny molecules of varying character. From a chemical point of view, some of them are reminiscent of the stress hormone cortisol and the sex hormones oestrogen, progesterone and testosterone, the so called steroid hormones.

Pheromones are transported in the air from one individual to another and reach the receiving person through the nose. Inside the nose, the so-called vomeronasal organ reacts to pheromones and activates the older areas of the brain. Pheromones therefore influence us at a subconscious level. It is not yet fully understood whether pheromones affect us humans via the ancient vomeronasal organ or via the nasal mucosa. Still, if we become attracted to someone or feel repugnance for them, or if we become calm or anxious, it may be due to the pheromones that someone is sending out that affect our brain in different ways.

Love at first sight

The child's closeness and searching behaviour after the birth help to reinforce the parents' love for the child and the desire to look after it, give it food and warmth and protection. The desire or instinct to get close to each other is there, but the details of the behaviour are formed in the meeting between the parents and the child through different sensory impressions – touch, warmth, pressure, sound and the sight of each other – which shape and further develop the innate behaviour.

Anxiety, alertness and aggression

A new mother is usually calmer than usual, especially when she has her child with her, but she can also become more vigilant, anxious and tense in certain situations. She is also protecting her child. She keeps a close eye on the surroundings and should anything or anyone threaten her child, she would jump to its defence and she will have access to unimaginable powers.

But the mother's anxiety can also be more diffuse. Suddenly, she might feel uncomfortable to leave her home, to meet unfamiliar people, to drive the car, go over bridges or watch TV programmes on violence. In addition, mothers can become enormously powerful and aggressive if someone threatens their child, the equivalent of the 'maternal aggression' seen in other mammalian mothers'

On an evolutionary level it is, of course, about the mother avoiding risks during the time that she is still vulnerable and the child is unable to manage on its own. She will need to defend herself and the child from various dangers. This unconscious caution and propensity for defence have probably saved many children in the early history of humans, and although we live in a much more protected world today, these reactions remain as a part of our mammalian heritage.

For some mothers, these worry reactions dominate; vigilance takes over and they have trouble sleeping, get anxious, become depressed and are in need of professional help. Of course, a strong emotional bond also affects the mother's priorities and choices. For many, the working career feels less important and it is about finding a balance between how much you want to be away from home and what is necessary for the professional life and the family income. But that is another book and another story.

Breastfeeding

When a mother is breastfeeding her child, nerve impulses are activated which are transmitted via the spinal cord to the supraoptic and paraventricular nuclei in the hypothalamus where oxytocin is formed. Due to the strong stimulation, the oxytocin-producing cells begin to operate as one single unit and not as a number of individual cells. Then, when all of the oxytocin cells are simultaneously activated, which occurs approximately in 90-second intervals, a pulse of oxytocin is delivered into the bloodstream from the dosal lobe of the pituitary and with each pulse of oxytocin, the muscles in the milk containers in the breast contract to cause a let-down of milk.

Through nerves, oxytocin also reaches down into the anterior lobe of the pituitary gland, where it stimulates the release of prolactin, which is the most important hormone for the production of milk. At the same time, the blood vessels in the front of the chest expand and the temperature increases. Both milk and warmth are thus transferred to the child.

Increased social interaction, calm and peace

But the mother is also affected in other ways. Since oxytocin is also released in the brain during each breastfeed, mothers become more interactive towards their child, more sensitive to its needs and also calmer during each feed. During the breastfeed, she also relaxes physically because her blood pressure drops and the level of the stress hormone, cortisol, decreases.

At the same time, the activity in her stomach and intestines increases so that she can digest, absorb and store nutrition in the most optimal way. During lactation, the mother is required to feel calm, sensitive and focused on her child but also nutritionally effective. One cannot give out energy without at the same time saving energy and this is precisely what happens when the muscle activity and stress-level decrease while the activity in the gastrointestinal tract and nutrient storage are increased.

The oxytocin-induced changes in maternal behaviour seen in lactation serve to strengthen the effects created by oxytocin release during childbirth. Breastfeeding may also, to some extent, compensate for and replace the lack of oxytocin in the brain during births where the mother had a Caesarean section or epidural anaesthesia.

Long-term effects of breastfeeding

In addition to making the mother calm and relaxed during each breastfeeding opportunity, the effect of oxytocin during lactation is more long lasting. The levels of the stress-related hormone cortisol are reduced between breastfeeds and the blood pressure becomes lower. This is because when oxytocin is released often such as during breastfeeding, it also affects the function of other signalling systems, thereby creating long-term beneficial effects.

The calming and relaxing effects can last for a very long time and may even protect women in the long term from certain stress-related illnesses later in life. It has, in fact, been shown in large clinical investigations that women who breastfeed are 'dose dependently' protected from certain cardiovascular diseases such as heart attacks, stroke and high blood pressure. This means that the more children they breastfeed and the longer that breastfeeding continues, the more protected they are. To some extent they are also protected against type 2 diabetes, the type of diabetes that occurs in adults or older people. This protection against certain stress-related illnesses, which has been observed in women who breastfeed, is probably due to the repeated oxytocin release that occurs during breastfeeding.

The role of skin-to-skin contact

We described earlier what happens when a newborn baby is placed on the mother's chest after the birth and how they seek contact with each other, becoming calmer and more relaxed. These effects happen because skin-to-skin contact triggers the oxytocin system, albeit not as much as breastfeeding does. Only certain parts of the oxytocin effect patterns operate during skin-to-skin contact. If you study the blood levels of oxytocin, you only see a few protracted pulses of oxytocin, and not the short pulses that occur at 90-second intervals in response to suckling. However, oxytocin is also released from some of the nerves in the brain that contain oxytocin. This contributes towards making the newborn feel good and safe, increases social interaction and lowers stress levels. The functions that support nutritional uptake and growth are also strengthened.

Touch and closeness are an important part of each breastfeed. In fact, most of the lactation-related changes have already started before the baby even begins to suckle while the baby is lying with the mother. She becomes calmer, and opens up to the child. She becomes more interactive and she relaxes as her blood pressure and cortisol levels start to drop. The baby is also affected by the skin-to-skin contact. The baby becomes calmer and the desire to interact with the mother and to feed is increased. But the milk is only released when the baby starts to suckle.

The kangaroo method

Many hospitals have now acknowledged the effectiveness of skin-to-skin contact and started to ensure that babies benefit from this closeness. We now know that babies who are born too early – so-called premature babies – thrive and grow better if they have skin-to-skin contact with their mother or father rather than being confined to an incubator.

The kangaroo method was 'discovered' by chance in Colombia in South America. The Colombians simply did not have the resources to take care of premature babies and had to find a workable solution. The South American babies were treated by turning a shawl into a kind of 'nest' at the mother's chest. This kind of treatment was called the 'kangaroo method' because it's reminiscent of a baby joey resting in its mother's pouch.

This method has been tested in many countries. Researchers have compared the development of premature babies who have been treated with the kangaroo method with babies treated in an incubator. The results show that the kangaroo babies, who got warmth and touch from their parents, put on more weight, developed faster and could leave the hospital earlier than the babies who were treated in an incubator. The mothers' milk production was also better.

The use of the kangaroo method is on the increase and the use of the method in the care of premature babies also has the benefit of allowing the father to participate in the treatment, which means his relationship with the child is more stimulated and he becomes more involved in the care.

The bond is strengthened

The American paediatrician, Marshall Klaus, has described how skin-to-skin contact between parents and children in early life leads to a strengthening of the bond between them. He found that mothers whose babies were placed in incubators behaved differently to mothers who had their babies with them on the maternity ward. New mothers are usually very attentive when a paediatrician examines their baby. But Marshall Klaus noted that mothers of premature babies often handed the baby over to the doctor and then went and sat down on a chair in another part of the room. He concluded that these mothers had not bonded with their child and developed their maternal behaviour to the same extent as mothers normally do.

More interested and intuitive parents

Klaus had a feeling that the 'deviant' behaviour of these mothers was caused by their separation from their babies. He, therefore, performed studies where he looked at the development of the relationship between the mother and the baby. He compared the interactions between mothers and babies that were separated from each other at birth and mothers who had received skin-to-skin contact with their baby at birth. He found that if the mothers had been allowed skin-to-skin contact with their baby, the bonding and attachment between the two developed quicker and breastfeeding worked better. The positive effects of the skin-to-skin contact after birth could be measured for weeks, months and perhaps even years later, even if the closeness only lasted a few hours.

His findings have been confirmed by other researchers who have shown that if the mother and baby have had close contact immediately after the birth (preferably skin-to-skin), the mother pays more attention to her baby, has an easier time understanding what it needs, smiles to it, looks into its eyes more often and talks to it in a way which is more suitable for a baby (motherese). In general, parents think that their own children are more beautiful than other children. This is particularly true when they have had close contact with their baby straight after the birth. Taken together all these data show that early closeness creates a stronger bond between the mother and baby. The baby also becomes more positive towards its mother and finds it easier to understand what she wants.

In Sweden, and in many other countries, fathers are often present at the birth and during the first few days thereafter. The fathers often have skin-to-skin contact with their babies during this time. What consequences might this have? Some studies have shown that the new age father has changed. Fathers have become softer and more considerate towards their families and are more likely to prioritise the family over their career. There are even studies that show that fathers who stay home to look after their children, which means a lot of closeness and skin-to-skin contact with them, have lower levels of the male hormone testosterone during this period!

The child is also affected by early closeness

At one year of age, a child who had close contact with its mother directly after birth is calmer and copes with stress better than a child who was separated from its mother. Both mother and child are also better at understanding each other and communicating with each other. That it really is the early skin-to-skin contact which enhances the connection between mother and child can be shown because clothes to some extent counteract the effect of the early closeness by functioning as an insulating layer.

As mentioned above, the ability to communicate, bond with others and become calm can be activated by a short moment of closeness early on in life. But this close contact between mother/father and child is not just important in those early days but also has lasting long-term implications. It is of course possible to create a good relationship later on in life, but it will take a longer time. It is as if early in life there is a 'free shot' – or in more technical terms a 'biological window' – to quickly establish a positive connection, which has implications for the ability to interact and deal with stress for a very long time to come.

There are, at the moment, no similar studies where the effect of early closeness has been looked at in children older than a year. But we know that a lot of closeness in connection with the birth and the early days of life decreases the risk of mothers abandoning their children. This was demonstrated in studies from both Russia and Thailand. It also seems that the tendency to abuse children is reduced.

On the other hand, there are many studies showing that early separation is not good, that children who are abandoned or who lost their loved ones very early in life fare less well. They might have problems with their physical health, such as difficulty in growing and combating infections. There are also many studies showing that they might have problems in their relationships and that they are at increased risk of suffering from anxiety and depression-related disorders. If you turn these results on their head, we could say that closeness to your loved ones when you're young protects against anxiety, depression and relationship problems in adulthood and may also promote your physical health.

Long-lasting effects

The fact that the oxytocin-related effects associated with childbirth and the time just after are long-lasting is probably because the oxytocin release is stronger at this time than at any other time in life. It has previously been mentioned that repeated oxytocin release produces long-lasting effects by influencing functions in other signalling systems. It is possible that the enormous amounts of oxytocin released in a short period of time during labour create the same kind of pattern that is seen when there is repeated oxytocin release over a longer time period. The unusually high levels of the pregnancy hormones, oestrogen and progesterone, together with the high stress level, including high cortisol levels, are also important in making the effects so powerful.

In addition, many other systems in the brain that facilitate learning shift into a higher gear during this period. The closeness immediately after the birth seems to have a particular ability to affect the child in the long term. It is possible that the activation of or switching off of certain genes (epigenetic programming of the type that Michael Meaney describes in young rats that receive a lot of closeness and nurturing early on in life, see Chapter 2) also occurs in humans.

Oxytocin in the brain mediates 'skin satisfaction'

According to the model of closeness presented in this book, and as Harry Harlow has pointed out, there is a certain 'skin hunger' which can only be satisfied by closeness. But what do we know about the regulation of skin hunger or the hunger of the skin? Not a lot, because this particular need has not been clearly defined physiologically. However, we can assume that such a primitive need as skin hunger, in the same manner as the need for food, is regulated in part in the hypothalamus.

We have previously described how closeness between, for example, a mother and a baby encourages social interaction, lowers anxiety, and creates a feeling of well-being and calm. Closeness also lowers stress levels and blood pressure, and increases nutritional uptake. We have shown that these effects are created by closeness because touch and warmth, and light pressure activate sensory nerves in the skin. We also described how the oxytocin release in the brain appeared to have an important co-ordinating function with regards to the patterns of effects created by closeness or the stimulation of sensory nerves from the skin. Finally, we have described how the administration of oxytocin produces precisely the effects that closeness or the stimulation of skin nerves gives rise to.

If we bring together the discussion about skin hunger with the information in the summary above, one could say that skin hunger is satisfied by the calming and relaxing effects that are created by oxytocin release induced when skin nerves are activated by warmth, touch and light pressure.

Secure attachment through oxytocin

Perhaps a secure child who received a lot of closeness from its parents has 'learnt or memorised' the experiences of the touch-induced effects of oxytocin in the brain more efficiently and in fact even developed a higher activity in its oxytocin system than less secure children. If so, this effect can be viewed from a further physiological perspective. As mentioned before, repeated oxytocin treatment gives rise to long-term, more or less, chronic effects via stimulation of the function in other signalling systems. In the child who receives a lot of good contact with its mother or father, the oxytocin system is activated repeatedly. Consequently the signalling system that regulates social competence and calm may be adapted by the released oxytocin towards increased social competence and reduced stress reactivity.

The fact that the children who get closeness via skin-to-skin contact immediately after birth and during the first hours that follow have a much better interaction with their mothers at the age of one year, and are also calmer compared to those that did not have close contact could be explained by a facilitation or strengthening of the 'learning, memorisation or conditioning' of the touch-induced effects during this time period. Alternatively these effects could become life-long by switching certain genes on or off.

Relaxed from a distance

One can imagine that the child eventually associates its parents with well-being and calm. When the child is in close contact to its parents, sensory nerves of the skin are stimulated (especially on the front of the chest) from the warmth, pressure and touch, which releases oxytocin and contributes towards the child feeling well and becoming calm.

At the same time as the sensory nerves are stimulated, triggering calm and relaxation, the child sees and hears the parents as many senses are active at the same time. Eventually, the child doesn't need to be physically near its parent; it is enough to see or hear the parent to make the child feel good and experience calm and peace. The sight or sound of the parent has then become linked to the release of oxytocin and the effects that the sensory stimulation triggers – a kind of Pavlovian conditioning has been created. A similar reaction is triggered in the parents, who also become satisfied and reassured by having their children near. The conditioning works in both directions.

In the next phase of the development, the parents don't need to be in the same room because the child has created a memory or an inner picture of them which they keep in their head. It's enough to think about their mother or father to become calm. In the older child the skin hunger resurfaces especially when the child feels a bit worried. At this point, the purely mental effects from the calming inner picture of its mother are not enough but the picture needs to be reinforced by the more basic activation of the sensory nerves from the skin for the child to overcome the fear. To curl up in mum's or dad's lap or to receive a hug does the trick.

At best, the learned calm created by the early closeness lasts for a lifetime. It can also be further developed to become more universal and triggered by many other people who seem secure and trustworthy. The person who first activated the calm and peace system does not need to be present; she or he is in the memory as a learned image and has a decisive significance on the child's security and ways of functioning later in life.

In support of the view that oxytocin has a central role in the development of attachment it can be mentioned that several studies show that children's oxytocin levels correlate positively with secure attachment. Even in older children, their oxytocin levels reflect how secure they are. Further evidence of the connection between oxytocin, a good relationship with the mother and secure attachment is seen in Romania. It was found that some children raised in orphanages, who did not receive enough closeness when they were small, were unable to release oxytocin later in life when they met people that they liked, in contrast with their peers who had received normal closeness with adults when they were young.

The mother is not covered in the Bowlby model

Oxytocin creates a bond between mother and child in the same way as in other mammals, which means that they feel good and calm when they are together. If a new mother leaves her child, she can therefore easily become anxious. Even this feeling can be connected to oxytocin and is in mammalian language a signal to the mother to return to her child. Oxytocin thus contributes to 'sticking together' mother and child because worry and tension is dispersed when they are together.

A key difference between Bowlby's model of care and the closeness model described here is that Bowlby related the mother's nurturing of the child as a separate maternal behaviour. But it's not just the child that needs closeness; the reverse is also true. As I have described above, the mother also becomes positively affected by the closeness to the child; she feels happy, content and calm. According to this way of looking at things, the mother's maternal behaviour is activated by the oxytocin that is released in readiness during the birth and which is later amplified by the oxytocin that is created by the closeness immediately after birth and by breastfeeding and closeness later on. The mother's skin hunger is brought to life through the oxytocin. The closeness of her child makes her feel good and relaxed. Equally she will suffer and become anxious when they are separated. Mother and child mirror each other.

Religion – a model of bonding?

When the small child grows up, gradually the relationship with the mother and other adults develops. An important aspect of this is that the child becomes secure and can display trust towards the mother, father or significant others. In the beginning, the child needs body contact to feel calm and secure but eventually it is enough that the parents are in the same room to trigger the safety system. At a later stage, the child will have 'internalised' the parent, in other words, she or he exists inside the head all the time and the child can feel calm and secure even when the parents are away. A small cute and furry teddy bear to hold can help to maintain the picture or positive feelings of the bond to the mother in the transitional period. The child will later add more safety figures, perhaps grandparents or a teacher at nursery or school. But all these figures have the limitation that they cannot always be present.

Here, for some people a religion such as Christianity provides an alternative solution to the problem. Even if God is not in the room, he's always present in heaven. He loves the children, as the prayer says and he sees them and holds them, just like the mother did in the beginning. It is as if the hymns and prayers help the children to create an additional attachment figure – someone who can always be present, perhaps not always in the room but in heaven.

What is all this if not the description of a beloved parent, mother or father or another loved one? Since God is an internal image you have to imagine him. The words in the prayers and hymns help to establish an image of the kind man in heaven. But it is the case with all relationships that they need nutrition to survive. By reading prayers every night and maybe singing hymns at regular intervals, you can keep the relationship with God alive.

At the same time as keeping the relationship alive, the person's own calm and security are increased, partly as a direct effect of the symbolic words that describe love, calm and security, but also indirectly because the image of the kind god, who constantly thinks of the children, sees them and holds them, becomes more vivid. Moreover, God has his own houses on earth, namely the churches, and here and in other places there are pictures of the kind man who lives in heaven.

This also helps us reinforce the image of God and the feeling of being enclosed and secure that he creates. The prayer is also a kind of conversation with God. The children's kind god is a substitute good parent or perhaps more likely a granddad.

The need to expand our safety system remains throughout life. It is not just the children who need it. For the adults who have a personal relationship with the kind god, this could be the source of all the above-described positive feelings and experiences in life. It would be like always having someone's hand to hold, always feeling secure and never being alone, because someone always sees you, hears you, and warms and holds you. Prayer and hymns may also contribute to relaxation and meditative feelings, which of course are also healthy and wholesome.

Monks and nuns who live in monasteries probably live in an extreme oxytocin world. The relationship with God is at the centre throughout the day. Regular mass and song maintain the relationship to the divine and the positive feelings that this brings. The regularity and the short interval between the masses and prayers mean that the oxytocin system is constantly running.

6

Oxytocin in adult relationships

A very important effect of oxytocin is its ability to stimulate different kinds of social interactive behaviours. We have already described how oxytocin activates the mammalian mother's nurturing of and relationship with her offspring. In this chapter we will show how oxytocin facilitates our relationships in adult life in a similar way.

Positive effects

Oxytocin, as mentioned, has the capability to diminish anxiety and fear. Administration of oxytocin reduces the fear that may be induced when meeting strangers or unfamiliar individuals. At the same time, social behaviours are stimulated, partly because the propensity to interact with other individuals is increased by oxytocin triggering different types of communicative behaviours. It may be through the sounds, smells or movement patterns. Oxytocin also increases the ability to interpret the nuances or emotional messages in communicative signals from other individuals.

Learning and association

Oxytocin also increases in particular an individual's ability to recognise other individuals as the learning or creation of a memory occurs more quickly. This effect has been demonstrated in experiments with rats. If a rat is treated with oxytocin prior to a first meeting with an unfamiliar rat, the oxytocin-treated rat is not afraid of the stranger. Nor is the oxytocin-treated rat afraid of this other rat at subsequent meetings. Not only the features of the unfamiliar rat but also the calming effect created by the oxytocin injection in connection with the first encounter are memorised and become associated with the other rat.

Reward, calm and peace

Oxytocin can create a number of effects that are perceived as pleasant. The activity in the brain's reward system can be stimulated which creates a feeling of well-being via an increase in the release of endogenous opioids and dopamine. The experience of pain is also subdued. The production of serotonin, which is linked to good mood, may increase and the production of the stress hormone cortisol is reduced because the activity in the HPA axis slows down. Other manifestations of stress, such as high blood pressure, can also be suppressed by a reduced activity in the sympathetic nervous system and the pulse slows down because the activity in the parasympathetic system increases.

All of these changes are most likely experienced as positive or even enjoyable. As these effects can be triggered by oxytocin release in connection with interactions with another individual

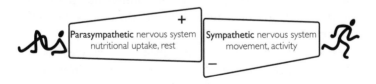

Illustration showing that oxytocin, in principle, increases the function of the parasympathetic nervous system and decreases the function of the sympathetic nervous system.

(it could be closeness between mother and offspring, or the sensory stimulation when a male and female mate, or the scent signals in a herd) the experience of the interaction becomes positive. If you keep close to the other person, the positive effects can be kept alive. But if you are separated from or leave the other individual, the positive effects fade and, in order to feel good again, you need to reunite with the other individual, for example, the mother with her child or the partner with his or her mate or the other animals in a herd. In this way, oxytocin ensures that individuals stay together.

Relationships in mammals

In the US, Thomas Insel and Sue Carter have shown how oxytocin facilitates the bonding or attachment between voles living in couple relationships. Normally, the strong bond between the female vole and the male vole is created by the release of oxytocin when they mate (in males vasopressin also plays an important role). During this time, they bond with each other. But if you administer oxytocin to the voles that have not yet formed a couple relationship while they have a vole of the opposite sex in front of them, they will bond without the need to mate.

There are several reasons for this 'unconscious' life-long choice of partner which occurs when the pair-living voles mate or have oxytocin administered. The oxytocin-affected individual can more easily recognise the other one and becomes less afraid of it. In addition, the vole's reward system is activated – substances such as dopamine and endorphins are released by oxytocin and this makes the other vole appear pleasant.

Finally, the animals become calm and relaxed as the calm and peace system that is activated by the administered oxytocin begins to take effect. Overall, this means that the voles continue to prefer the animal that they recognise and which has become associated with the positive experiences. Note that it is the same 'basic pattern' of effects that is created by oxytocin in the pair-living animals as in the relationship between mothers and their offspring.

It appears in the male vole that vasopressin, the relative of oxytocin, plays an important role in conjunction with oxytocin in promoting bonding with the female. It has even been shown that there are two kinds of vasopressin receptors, one long and one short. The long type appears to be linked to faithfulness and the other to a more promiscuous lifestyle, and one of them is present in voles living as pairs and the other in male voles who live in more harem-like groups.

In addition to the different types of vasopressin receptors, the localisation of oxytocin and vasopressin receptors in the brain is different between the voles living in pairs and the voles living in groups. It is not usually possible to create a bond between the voles that normally don't live as a pair but instead live in harem-like groups. However, it is possible to change the behaviour of the two types of voles with the use of modern techniques whereby genetic information is transferred from one type of vole to the other.

Sex and love

For most people the family becomes less important when they fall in love and find a partner they want to settle down with. The need for touch and closeness reduces as the child reaches adulthood, but then comes back when in a sexual relationship and becomes a very significant part of the communication between the couple. Next to childbirth and breastfeeding, sex is the most powerful trigger of oxytocin release. The touching and the kisses, but also the sensory stimulation of intercourse in itself, lead to high oxytocin release in both men and women.

There are studies in which researchers have measured the oxytocin level in men and women during sexual intercourse and they have found that the oxytocin level rises and reaches a maximum at the time of orgasm. Oxytocin might have many functions in this context. One effect is that the muscles that are involved in orgasm in men and women contract. From other studies it has been concluded that transportation of the egg and the fertilisation of the egg is made easier when the oxytocin levels are high.

Because oxytocin triggers the release of dopamine and endogenous opiates it can also contribute towards the well-being and happy feelings that are experienced in connection with intercourse and orgasm. The calm and peace and feelings of love and trust to the loved one could in the same way be connected to oxytocin. It has recently been shown that the calm that follows when rats have mated totally disappears if the animals are treated with substances that block the effects of oxytocin. The strong bond that arises between the two lovers is, of course, also down to oxytocin.

It is of course not only oxytocin that is in charge and playing havoc with our bodies when we are in love and perhaps lose our heads a bit. There are studies which show that an amphetamine-like substance is created in the brain during this falling in love period which can actually last for years. It has also been shown that serotonin levels fall in the couple in love, perhaps as an expression of their need to be close to each other to feel really good. Low levels of serotonin are usually connected to hunger and aggression, but in this case it is a hunger for the loved one, a type of 'skin hunger'.

Sexuality is often enhanced in women who are in love. This has been connected to increased levels of the male hormone testosterone which in women drives sexuality. However, in men the opposite is true! Their testosterone levels decrease, which can contribute to or be caused by the increased closeness to the loved one.

The fact that touch and closeness can play a big part in lowering testosterone levels is supported by the findings that testosterone levels also decrease in fathers who stay at home with their children. In the same way as the contact between the parents and the child, the body contact becomes more pleasant in couples in love. As part of the erotic attraction a skin hunger is 'resurrected' as an important pulling power between them.

The skin becomes so to speak 'charged and electric'.

When the loved ones are close to each other they feel good, they become calm and relaxed. But when they are apart, this well-being and calmness disappears and they want to see each other again. As time goes on, these pleasant and calming effects are connected to the other person, even if the individual is not present apart from in the world of thoughts. This is exactly the same development as seen in parents and children. It becomes unbearable not to be close to each other.

The same mechanisms as in the parent-child relationship

There are many similarities between the first meeting of a parent and child skin-to-skin after the birth and the intercourse between the two lovers. In both situations, two individuals become close in a relatively rule-conforming way. The preparation for breastfeeding is similar to the preparation for intercourse, and includes different types of sensory stimulations like touch, warmth, pressure and smells. Communications between the two adults often include small sounds similar to those that the mother and child use. For both parties the situation is connected to well-being and a feeling of being calm, relaxed and happy.

In the breastfeeding mother, the oxytocin release can be so strong that she experiences being in her own world. The level of consciousness can also become decreased during intercourse. Afterwards, both might go to sleep.

Mother and child, the couple in love, and indeed all individuals who like each other, feel happiness and contentment when they meet or think about each other. It is possible with the use of fMRI to show how the areas in the brain which are associated with strong positive emotions and which are connected to oxytocin light up both in the mother when she sees a picture of her beloved child and in the couple in love when they see pictures of each other.

If the lovers are allowed to be close to each other when the oxytocin level is high, the same process takes place as when the parents and a newborn baby meet. The body's reward system is stimulated and the person and the surrounding environment are coloured by one's own oxytocin filter. The other party will similarly be linked to calm, relaxation and decreased anxiety. And just as the new parents find their own child more beautiful and wonderful than anyone else, the lovers perceive each other as perfect, partly due to their own oxytocin.

Destroyed boundaries in strong relationships

In people who are close to each other the 'boundaries' between them can partly be abolished. If you think about parents and children it is a given. It is apparent that the parents must take responsibility and take action to protect their children. When you think about adults it may seem absurd.

Nevertheless, it is basically the same mechanism which affects both parties because the strong influences of oxytocin increase the ability to be responsive to others' feelings and desires. The two individuals also tend to mimic each other. They mirror each other's facial expressions and feelings which also leads to a synchronisation of movements and to some extent, thoughts. Many people who have been married or lived together for a long time can, in the end, know what the other person is thinking without saying it. They can often read each other's thoughts. Sometimes two people who have been together for a long time start to look like each other. They have the same posture and facial expressions, and they become what is usually referred to as soul mates.

At a major international conference many years ago, I met a woman who was married to one of my research colleagues. It was obvious that they liked each other a lot. Although the wife had no research training and had never been in the laboratory, she referred to her husband's research as 'their' research. In her mind they had performed the work together. At the time, I thought what she was saying was absurd. Today, I look at the whole thing differently. She obviously perceived that she and her husband were in part the same person.

When lovers are separated

Before the mental picture of the other party has been properly established, the well-being and calm prevail more in the moment. But what happens when they are separated? Well, it is exactly the same feeling as for parents and children. If the beloved person is not close by, the pleasant feelings disperse after a while. You start to feel a bit anxious and nervous. 'Where is she?' 'Why doesn't he call?' 'Could she have met someone else?' Slowly, the bright world of thoughts is exchanged for a dark hole of concern.

What is this? Well, it's the opposite side of bonding or attachment as previously described in connection with the parent-child relationship; the part connected to abandonment, anxiety and vigilance. The point of attachment is that the two people should be together, and they are simply held together by an invisible mooring. In the same way that the parent and the child become anxious after a time of separation, the two people in love become anxious and may experience deep despair and worry when they are separated, especially at the beginning of the relationship, before the inner mental picture has been firmly fixed and they trust each other.

There are researchers who claim that women are more sensitive to the downsides of separation and therefore may suffer more in less established relationships where feelings still exist. The wonderful nights are followed by days of abandonment, deep despair and anxiety. This biological phenomenon reoccurs after each meeting and won't disappear unless the relationship becomes of a more permanent character. The reaction is probably an expression of the underlying cohesive forces in a relationship. It doesn't matter how enlightened and liberated we are, we are unable to access these primordial reactions which is more of an expression of our mammalian heritage.

Love and bonding – not always a parallel

This invisible negative aspect of bonding or attachment may partly explain some experiences and observations that may seem difficult to understand. The various aspects of the connecting strings in a relationship do not always run in parallel with each other. Love may fade and one of a pair may no longer be interested. Sometimes there might even be hints of threats and violence. And still, the couple stay together. To an outsider, it may seem inconceivable that the two do not separate and that the abandoned or abused doesn't break up the relationship.

There may be many reasons why a person chooses to remain in a difficult or eventually dangerous relationship. It can be about practical things such as economy, housing and the custody of the children. But in addition, it may be that a deep need for security lives on and the partner is still able to fulfil this need, even if the love has died and it would be better to end the relationship.

A learned (conditioned) security response is not so easy to erase because these links between the two individuals lie in very deep areas of the personality. Paradoxically, it may, therefore, feel both anxious and agonising to separate from someone whom you do not like. The time alone is not only relief, but also a period filled with incomprehensible anxiety and worry. During this time, the invisible belt may bring the couple back together and reconciliation and reunification lead to a temporary relief. And this can happen again and again. It may take a long time for the invisible tie to loosen.

The strong bond – a support for change

The tie between two lovers is very strong, not least because oxytocin is released in large quantities during lovemaking, but also through kisses and caressing. The bond that held together the herd or group in mankind's childhood was also incredibly strong. It was probably very difficult to leave the group. In order to do so, an even stronger bond was probably needed, such as being in love. We didn't live very long so it was important to find a partner and have children at a young age. Perhaps this is why the bond between man and woman becomes especially strong if created at a young age?

Today, we don't always live in such life-long relationships. Many people marry and divorce or have many different relationships throughout their lives. But there are many people who are unexpectedly reunited with their first love in later life, and these relationships often flourish and the couple live happily for many years. There seems to be something special about these early relationships.

Love on the phone

People who like each other look into each other's eyes often and perhaps also speak to each other with a soft and playful voice. They also smile a lot at each other. This occurs both in a mother and child relationship and when a couple are in love. However, the two grown-ups in love don't always have to be in the same room to express their feelings; they can also use the telephone. In that case, it's the words and the tone of voice that express the message of love, and that works well too. Oxytocin does not only make our faces friendly and inviting, the voice also reveals our feelings.

The spoken words express emotion and the 'voice' in the other receiver listens and answers with a similar tone of voice. The other partner is 'indirectly present' because the two of them create an inner picture of each other. The presence of a human is in this way replaced by the inner picture of the other individual, who can therefore be in a completely different location. In some relationships, the telephone can be a very important link for a very long time.

Before the telephone, letters had to work as the link between the separated couple though they are not as direct as a face-to-face meeting or a meeting on the phone. On the other hand, the written word is less evasive and the letters could be read over and over again.

Today the internet has become an important tool for relationships. Matchmaking seems to occur over the net and also long-term correspondence between friends and lovers. In this case the mental image or memory of 'the other', and not the face, the voice or even the handwriting, will be responsible for the emotional interpretation of the messages. This is not always easy and may of course lead to serious misinterpretations.

Oxytocin and friendship

As we have seen, oxytocin has a number of effects apart from the classical effects during childbirth and breastfeeding. These take place in the brain through the release of oxytocin from nerves, though the oxytocin can also reach important regulating areas in the brain in other ways. Oxytocin also works by activating other signalling systems which, in turn, start processes which can:

- Reduce fear
- Stimulate social behaviour
- Facilitate interpretation of 'communicative signals' (for example through smell, hearing and sight)
- Facilitate recognition and bonding
- Create well-being
- Create calm and trust
- Reduce the sensations of pain
- Reduce the release of stress hormones
- Lower pulse and blood pressure
- Stimulate nutritional uptake, growth and healing.

You could look at the oxytocin-mediated effects from a larger perspective. In the same way that dangerous and uncomfortable contacts with the skin can cause the protective fight-and-flight response or a calm-and-peace response depending on the type of stimulation, experiences through other senses, like odour, hearing and sight, can cause different patterns of response depending on the value of the sensory experience. Added to this, our inner pictures, which are created by 'moving in' memories from external experiences, also cause such responses. If the inner or outer experience is understood as safe, warm and touching, for example a meeting with another human, oxytocin is released and in this way the oxytocin effects are created which increase social interaction, reduce fear, decrease anxiety levels, and induce feelings of relaxation and calmness but also trust. The latter effects are communicated by the amygdala and the hippocampus complex, where unconscious judgements are made as to whether the environment should be perceived as dangerous or safe or even pleasant or attractive.

Oxytocin makes us more susceptible and responsive to impulses from the environment by decreasing the influence from the controlling frontal lobe in the brain cortex but it also creates bodily and mental effects of the friendly, calm and relaxing kind if the environment is judged to be warm, touching and supporting.

Friendship and warm relationships

You don't have to give birth, breastfeed or have a sexual relationship in order to gain access to the positive effects that warmth and support can create. In fact, these types of reaction are initiated in all people who interact on a positive and friendly level. The difference is that this occurs through touch or warmth or even other, more indirect forms of contact, especially through the experience of someone seeing, listening and supporting you.

The American researcher Kathy Light has shown that oxytocin is released in adult people who have close and warm contact with each other. Less oxytocin is released than during breastfeeding and intercourse. But it is enough for us to respond with joy and relaxation when we meet people with whom we experience a deep connection. The warm feelings are also accompanied by calm and relaxation, both physically and mentally.

Oxytocin stimulates social interaction in humans

With the use of the fMRI technique, it has been shown that after the administration of oxytocin via nasal spray to men several different parts of the human brain involved in social interaction are affected. This suggests that the administration of oxytocin reduces fear and increases social ability by working in many different areas in the brain, thereby producing a pattern of effects consistent with social interaction. This results in an increased ability to interpret other people's emotional state, in a more friendly and generous behaviour towards other people, and even in a more positive view of the world. In this way, positive circles are created.

In another study, men were asked to interpret facial expressions by being shown images of the area around other people's eyes. The illustrated eyes expressed different emotions, from anger to surprise and being in love. The men who had received oxytocin nasal spray were more often correct in assessing the state of mind that the picture showed compared with the control group who received a saline nasal spray. In a similar study, a group of men with autistic traits, who had difficulties being in contact with other people, were tested. These men also became better at interpreting the emotional content of the images.

A further study showed that oxytocin given through a drip into the bloodstream also influenced social skills in a positive way. Here, the experimental group, which consisted of men with autistic traits and who consequently had trouble interacting with other people, interpreted the emotional content of voices. They had to determine if the person talking was angry, friendly or scared. The men who received an oxytocin drip for a few hours were better at determining the emotion of the voice and this improvement seemed to persist for several weeks. The amount of oxytocin that was given to the men was of the same levels that women are given to stimulate the contractions during labour.

People who have problems both with recognition of other

people and difficulties in interpreting their emotions and feelings often have low levels of oxytocin or a reduced ability to respond to oxytocin due to insensitivity of the oxytocin receptors. The results of all these studies show that oxytocin is of importance for social abilities in humans.

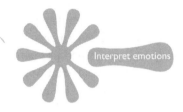

It is likely that some people whom we perceive as particularly nice and generous increase our own oxytocin levels and thus make us more interactive, calm and trusting. Oxytocin makes us more trusting without us knowing it because these reactions belong to our mammalian heritage and therefore take place on an unconscious level.

The group and the herd

When the mammalian offspring have grown up and left their mothers, they enter into other types of relationships. The mammals can live in small and large herds and they can even live in pairs, although the latter is unusual; only around five per cent of all mammals do so. Either if the animals live in a pair or in a larger group, oxytocin appears to play an important role for the interaction amongst and the cohesion between the various members of the group or the pair. Oxytocin exerts all these different effects by triggering and co-ordinating effects in other signalling systems. From a basic perspective this resembles the effect pattern that oxytocin exerts in the relationship between mothers and children.

Outside of the protection of the group, the lonely individual lives dangerously, almost like the newborn offspring who strays from its mother. During evolution, therefore, a variety of physical and behavioural adaptations developed to enable unity. One of the prerequisites for a group to stick together is that the different individuals recognise each other. They must also be able to read others' emotional states and then act accordingly.

The British researcher Barry Keverne has pointed out that certain areas in the brain related to recognition and social skills are particularly well developed in mammals that live in herds or packs. There are even correlations between the size of these parts of the brain and the number of individuals in the group.

Activation of the reward system

But it's not enough that the different individuals in the group recognise each other, can determine the other members' moods and that they are not afraid of each other for the group to keep together. The mechanisms that bond mother and child or adult couples also function as invisible glue in larger groups, although the intensity of the reactions is less pronounced.

There is research evidence which shows that morphine-like substances are released when monkeys groom each other's fur. The grooming is actually a way of keeping the pack together because it creates well-being in the one who gets groomed, and also in the one who grooms. This effect is probably related to the ability of touch and oxytocin to stimulate the body's reward system. In addition stress levels are decreased by grooming which contributes to the wish of the individuals to stay together.

The calming and unifying effects need not necessarily be mediated via closeness. Sight and sound certainly contribute as well. In addition, the signals between the different members of a group or a pack may be mediated through pheromones. Pheromones are, as we've seen earlier, airborne substances transferring from one individual to another and then affecting the receiving individual via an effect in the olfactory organ and the vomeronasal organ.

The animals become more social

The administration of oxytocin affects the social behaviour of animals in groups. If several animals (rats, for example) are brought together, they fight less if they are given oxytocin. They also sit closer together and sometimes they groom each other (and sometimes themselves).

If a lonely rat receives oxytocin it becomes, in some tests, a little bit bolder. It ventures, for example, to the middle of the cage, which is something that rats wouldn't normally do because it could be dangerous. The decreased fear is probably part of, or even a supposition for, the increase in social behaviour. A frightened or 'shy' rat does not approach other animals unless it intends to fight to determine who is the strongest and thus the leader of the group.

The reduced fear and increased social behaviour are created by oxytocin in the amygdala, the area of the brain which is of great importance for the regulation of anxiety and social interaction. Rats and mice that lack oxytocin or oxytocin receptors in the amygdala lose their ability to learn to recognise their own species and thus also to socialise with them in a normal way. In a sense these rats become 'autistic'.

In one series of experiments with rats it has been shown that if an individual animal receives administered oxytocin, not only does the rat itself become calm and more interactive towards the other rats but also all the rats who are in the immediate surroundings behave in the same way, and this happens without any touching. This is partly because rats with high levels of oxytocin secrete pheromones. The recipient animals thus become calmer and more interactive through the airborne substances that affect the olfactory organ, an effect that disappears if the nasal mucosa of the animal is anaesthetised. The animals exposed to pheromones also become less stressed and less susceptible to pain.

The effects that the odour signals give rise to in the other rats are the typical effects associated with oxytocin, and indeed the pheromones increase the release of oxytocin in the recipient rats. In this way, a kind of oxytocin level synchronisation happens in the group, which leads to the group as a whole becoming calmer and the individual animals interacting in a non-violent way with each other. They probably feel good too.

Just as the mother and child create well-being and calm in each other through touch, this process takes place in the rat group by the sending out of olfactory signals. But the rats need to stick to the group where the olfactory signals are, because if one of the odour-affected animals leaves the group, the positive oxytocin effects will subside along with the feelings of well-being and tranquillity. The rat would need to go back to its peers in the group to feel good again. In this way, the group is held together by the recognition of each other's scent and also because the olfactory signals activate the oxytocin system in the other members of the group. It is important to point out that the animals in a group are kind towards each other, but not necessarily towards animals in other groups. Animals in a foreign group are more likely to be met with increased suspicion and aggression.

The spreading of the calming effect is accelerated because the animals with higher oxytocin levels are attractive. Because the animals with high oxytocin levels attract the other animals, the recipient animals become more easily influenced by the olfactory signals that the oxytocin-packed animals emit, and this further strengthens the unity of the group. The bonding in the group will naturally not be as specific as between mother and baby or between the two in a pair, but is more diluted and directed towards many individuals, almost like the many strings in a bunch of balloons.

People with experience of cows and cow management have observed that the barn will be very calm when a cow is about to give birth. The other cows lie down, ruminate and become generally peaceful. Perhaps the labouring cow, which of course has very high oxytocin levels, sends out high amounts of soothing scents which influence the release of oxytocin in other cows.

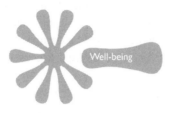

The modern group

Our *Homo sapiens* ancestors probably lived in groups of 50 to 60 individuals. They roamed around Africa and lived by hunting small animals and eating whatever grew in the trees and on the ground. They were hunters and gatherers who were continuously on the move, because they were not cultivating the land. It is reasonable to believe that some of our intuitive, innate talents were more important to our early ancestors than they are for us today, and that they were ruled by the 'mammalian heritage' to an even greater extent than us contemporary humans.

The cohesion and unity of the group must have been incredibly important because it was vital to protect and defend oneself against many dangerous animals and other unknown dangers. A good unity and co-ordination between individuals was obviously necessary with regards to hunting together or the defending of the group or clan.

Groups are, as mentioned earlier, held together with a kind of 'mini-oxytocin binder'. The rats in a group can soothe each other through oxytocin-linked pheromones, and other animals create positive unifying experiences by touching each other. These bonds are not as personal and unique as the bond between mother and child or in a pair relationship; they are more targeted towards all the individuals in the group. We humans are not as dependent on olfactory signals as some mammals but we recognise each other's appearance.

We no longer live in herds but we do spend much of our time in other types of groups, for example, in our workplace. Many employers also recognise the importance of reinforcing the sense of community among their employees. This will make them feel better and increase the chances that they will become loyal and work towards a common goal. Conference trips and various forms of 'events' are used to increase the unity of the group.

The power of the group bond is particularly noticeable when the unity ceases. Many people, after spending a week away from home on a stimulating course, will have experienced a feeling of emptiness when they return home and life returns to normal. This is nothing else other than a mild form of withdrawal symptoms or separation anxiety, showing that the unifying and positive effects of oxytocin were active only as long as the course lasted.

Us and the others

There are reasons to point out that there might be a downside to strong group bonds. In the same way that a strong interrelated couple can create a boundary towards the outside world, a unified group can do so too. A strong sense of 'us' feelings can be matched by a strong sense of 'the others' feelings. This 'us' against 'others' mentality is good when creating a team spirit to win a competition or working towards a common goal. On the other hand, a strong sense of group unity and the glue that this creates between the various members could be the cause of antagonism and even discrimination of various kinds between different groups.

The closer the individuals become and the more they lose the boundaries between themselves, the stronger the boundaries become outwards. It is as though there is a small shell that separates them from the outside world. It becomes 'us' and 'the others'. At the same time, one only sees the good and positive characteristics of members of the group, whereas negative traits are ascribed to outsiders. If this phenomenon is used incorrectly, alienation might become emphasised more than togetherness.

This tendency to perceive the world around us as 'us' and 'them', which is closely associated with the mechanisms that create bonds between individuals, can have a negative side because it can be an unconscious seed from which conflict grows.

The group and its ability to influence the oxytocin system is also used in various group therapeutic contexts. The security and trust that is created by being part of a group can provide the opportunity for major changes within the individual which they would never manage on their own.

7

Oxytocin and trust

Oxytocin is released by many different types of positive and warm encounters. When oxytocin is flowing, both parties become calm and they trust each other. We have previously described how important it is not to be afraid of other people when relating to them. A further aspect of the reduced fear is that you also trust other people. Trust is an important aspect of relationships.

Experiments have shown that trust is triggered by oxytocin. Marcus Heinrichs and his colleague Ernst Fehr did a study in which they administered oxytocin to men via a nasal spray. They showed that the men who received the oxytocin spray had greater trust in other people. The men had to play a computer game where they had to make money by investing a reasonable amount of money. The game included having to rely on a team-mate. Those men who had been treated with oxytocin showed a greater trust in their teammates than those treated with saline spray and they invested more money. Those who had participated in the study were informed of the outcome and what the study was about before they participated in a second study. Despite this information, those who received oxytocin spray became more trusting than those who didn't. This shows that one cannot affect trust just by will as trust occurs on an unconscious level.

Inner closeness

The stronger type of oxytocin release that occurs in the relationship between a mother and child and between two lovers eventually leads to an 'unconditional' bond between the two. In this way, the two individuals merge together, not just for the moment but also in the long run. However, oxytocin which is released in any other positive and warm closeness also creates a kind of bond between the individuals. These ties may not be as strong but they still contribute towards a feeling of unity and security.

When two or more individuals have bonded to each other, oxytocin is no longer released just by the physical closeness between the individuals. The initial closeness-related oxytocin release has become 'mentalised' and is awakened by the sight or thought of the other individual. Oxytocin is released via this 'internal closeness', and this activates the oxytocin-associated effect pattern. One could also say that the oxytocin release has been learned and that the oxytocin-mediated effects have been conditioned to the sight or mere thought of the other person, which, in a way, becomes ever present. This means that you feel good, become friendly towards others and calm in this type of 'internal meeting'. Once the bond has been created, the oxytocin effects, and thus trust, become more of a permanent fixture. You get an inner closeness.

Trusting or uncritical?

We tend to trust the person that we are closely bonded to and perhaps love. As a rule, this is obviously a prerequisite for a relationship to work. Oxytocin plays an important role in creating trust in those individuals who are exposed to high levels of oxytocin. But the high levels of oxytocin can also make the couple or group uncritical towards each other.

We sometimes say that love is blind and with modern techniques; it has actually been shown that areas in the brain which are related to critical thinking are 'turned off' in a mother who sees a picture of her child. The same thing happens when a person in love sees a picture of their partner.

When the system of trust is shaken up

It is essential that a mother and child or a couple in love have a mutual sense of trust. One consequence of trusting is that the information that is exchanged between them is accepted without question. Kind and positive statements can produce an amazing effect. But what happens if the person you love says something that is not nice or even perhaps something malicious or deceitful? The sad fact is that this, too, whether expressed in words or deeds, goes straight to the heart and hurts a lot. The person who loves can be mortally wounded by the beloved precisely because the openness to the other is so great.

When you lose a loved person, the oxytocin bond breaks and this hurts a lot. The pain may resemble that which is produced by normal physical wounds and may even be located in front of the body where the umbilical cord was once attached. At the same time, the inflow of relaxing positive effects that the closeness and presence of the loved person gave you comes to an end. Many people who have lost someone that they loved and lived with for a long time also become ill, and the risk of developing certain diseases, such as cardiovascular diseases, is increased.

You then need to be comforted and reassured so that the feelings of hurt, sadness, sorrow and pain may be expressed and you eventually come to terms with the loss. Once again, the touch and closeness from people who hold and comfort you will provide the best remedy. Perhaps the touch-released oxytocin softens not only the physical but also the mental pain when you are held and comforted? In fact, it has been shown that the same area in the brain is activated whether you have physical pain or mental pain. In grieving there is also an openness to the new, and it is not uncommon for a new love to emerge during this period. It is said that love heals all wounds.

It is as if the openness created by oxytocin also facilitates change and reconciliation, and thus creates possibilities for a continued life.

Deliberate manipulation of the trust system

To be betrayed by the one you love is of course a trauma that creates a great deal of suffering. But it's actually not only about the grief and the loss of a person but also about something much deeper. Your basic sense of security and confidence in the world can be shaken because oxytocin is so strongly associated with trust. In other words, basic security turns into distrust, suspicion and insecurity.

This vulnerability – being bonded or attached to certain individuals – can be used during times of war. Since one's trust, security, well-being, calm and ability to handle stress are linked to related individuals through the 'oxytocin-bond', most of us 'from the evil one's point of view' carry a weakness. By creating situations where the near and dear feel threatened for their health and life, or where the trust in those closest to us is shaken, you can get anyone side-tracked.

The trust systems are established early on in life

If the memory of betrayal and other unpleasant things are very deep rooted and they have been created early on in life, they can serve as barriers to all future close relationships. Some people have positive memories of their early relationships very strongly imprinted in their unconscious memory bank and others have more negative experiences. The inner pictures are important for how we respond to and manage the world around us. A kind and secure childhood, with much warmth and care, tends to make the inner picture nice and social, while the individual becomes calmer, more trusting and less afraid. A childhood marked by separations, threats and violence creates a more aggressive and fearful inner picture which of course influences the individual in all phases of life. These early experiences have an effect on whether one interprets events in a positive or negative way, and impact on the person's ability to trust or distrust other people.

Trust and strangers

A phenomenon which we have briefly touched on is that some people, regardless of the situation, seem to have the ability to more or less spread kindness, warmth and security to their fellow men. One possibility is that these individuals actually have higher levels of oxytocin, which is communicated to the surroundings in various ways.

One could imagine that oxytocin-packed people give off pheromones that stimulate oxytocin release in others, just like some mammals do, and that the olfactory signals could be part of the synchronisation of human emotions. It is said that you can smell fear; perhaps the same is true for calm. On the other hand, humans rely more on their vision and hearing when they assess their response to and their feelings towards other humans. It's important to study the body language, as well as the tone of voice. Most of all, however, we look at the face. What are the facial features? We pay extra attention to the area around the eyes. Here, one can actually see whether a person is kind, happy, angry or scared. There are a number of small muscles around the eyes over which we have only partial conscious control and the position of these muscles reflects our feelings.

Maybe the oxytocin-spreading humans look extra friendly, so friendly that even anxious and shy people in their vicinity become calmer and release their own oxytocin in response? People with a calm and friendly voice also have a great ability to calm and create unity. Perhaps this also affects other people's oxytocin release.

It is not always easy to prove such a rise in oxytocin in humans by measuring oxytocin levels in the blood as these effects take place in the brain. But, if one accepts that a friendly person can create such effects in other people, one may assume with a fairly high degree of probability that their oxytocin release has been activated and has affected certain areas of the brain. The calming person creates calm, reduced stress levels, relaxation, increased social communication and trust in others, which are precisely the effects created by the administration of oxytocin!

In most cases, we make a correct assessment when meeting a friendly person and we respond in kind. But there are some people who can turn on other people's oxytocin systems so that the 'victims' become trusting, kind and generous without themselves being affected. Conmen who cheat women out of money by a false promise of marriage belong to this group of people.

Trust when in need of help

There is another type of situation where trust can emerge and thus increase the susceptibility for positive impulses from another person, even if you don't know him or her particularly well. It is when you're in need of help. You may be unwell or otherwise in need of help and support. At this time, you're more likely to accept the touch from a stranger and let them cross your boundaries. Normally, you don't do this because it triggers your defence system.

There is a scientific study that shows that if a nurse holds the hand of a healthy person, the pulse and blood pressure increase. However, if that person is unwell and needs help, the pulse and blood pressure decrease. In the latter case, the closeness-related oxytocin reaction 'wins' against the defence mechanism because it is necessary to trust the person who helps when you are ill.

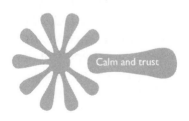

The Doula phenomenon

To explain how this works, we will look in a little more in detail at the so-called doula phenomenon, in other words how a supportive woman can facilitate and speed up a woman's labour. Women who give birth have through the ages looked for and received the help of other women. Childbirth originally used to take place in the home environment but at the beginning of the nineteenth century it began to move into hospitals. It was felt that it was safer to give birth where the experts and the technical equipment were and since then, childbirth has become something of a medical specialty.

The midwives still carry the practical primary responsibility but gynaecologists, anaesthetists and paediatricians are in close proximity at the hospital. Increasingly, various interventions are used during labour. Caesarean sections have become a common procedure, uterine contractions can be stimulated by oxytocin and the pain is muffled with pain medication or epidural anaesthesia.

The paediatricians, Marshall Klaus and John Kennell, noted during a trip to Guatemala that the births there, despite the lack of modern medical and technical aids, were quicker and easier than back home in the U.S. They naturally wondered how this could be and noted that, apart from the midwife, there were always one or more other women present during the births. It could be a relative or close friend. Perhaps it was the presence of these women which facilitated the entire birth process?

Back in the U.S., together with Phyllis Klaus, they conducted some research studies to investigate whether childbirth would become easier and faster if the women giving birth were accompanied by a female helper. They suggested that this helping woman should be called a doula, a word which they believed meant 'woman-helper' in Greek. (It turned out that the doula actually was the most important slave or servant in the Greek household in ancient times and they now wish they had chosen a different name.)

The studies showed that if a doula was present the births in the U.S. were quicker and that there were fewer complications. There were fewer Caesarean sections, and there was less of a need for an oxytocin drip to speed up labour, or to provide pain relief in the form of spinal anaesthesia or analgesic agents.

They also noticed that the mothers' experience of birthing was more positive and that they thought their children were the most beautiful in the world. Most new parents think so, but the fact is that the mothers who had the support of a doula were even more positive towards their newborn than those who didn't have access to a doula.

Even more surprising was that these trends lasted even after six weeks. The mothers still expressed greater self-esteem and security in their role of mothers and they were less depressed than the mothers who gave birth without a doula. Purely objectively, it was concluded that mother and child interacted better. The mothers also expressed themselves as being more positive about their husbands or partners.

Today, there are studies from several countries where it has been found that the presence of a doula during childbirth has a positive effect on the birth and the mother's relationship with her child. Naturally, the results vary depending on the country in which the studies were performed and the methods used, but basically all the studies show that the presence of another woman makes the birth easier and that the mother adapts better to the role of a mother.

How can it be that a relatively unknown woman can affect such diverse phenomena as how quickly the birth takes place, how easy the birth is and how well the mother gets along with her child and her husband? Well, the key to these effects is in the doula's physical and emotional support, which leads to an increase of activity in the mother's own oxytocin system. Paradoxically, an important prerequisite for this powerful effect is that the birthing woman is already influenced by her own oxytocin, as oxytocin is released during labour, and thus she is more trusting and willing to accept help from others.

First and foremost, the doula might hold the woman and

support her in a purely physical way. When she massages gently, she brings extra touch and warmth. But she is also present during the birth as emotional support. She listens to the needs of the mother and reassures her. She is compassionate and her continuous closeness creates peace and trust. She simply stimulates the mother's oxytocin release and increases her sensitivity to oxytocin by her closeness and presence.

Since the mother is open to help, an 'inner closeness' is created. The increase in the maternal oxytocin activity leads to the stress level being reduced so that the levels of stress hormones and the blood pressure don't become unnecessarily high. Because the mother is able to relax, it makes both the first stage of labour, when the cervix is opening up, and the pushing stage faster.

The increased activity in the oxytocin system also strengthens the mother's own pain relief. If the mother's experience of the birth is positive, this feeling is conveyed to the child, the father and all the others present at the birth. There are many doulas who can tell you how important they are in the new mother's life and how, for example, they are often invited to the child's birthdays for many years afterwards.

The doula effect – a universal phenomenon

The doula is thus a fellow being who, by support and touch and by her mere presence and her positive engagement, can make a woman give birth quicker by strengthening the effects of oxytocin on the uterus and other oxytocin effects such as those of a stress-reducing nature.

All people – men and women, young and old – also have oxytocin, not only in the blood but also in the brain. Why shouldn't human support trigger oxytocin effects in all individuals who need help? Maybe a calm, safe, touching and warm environment, in particular when it is embodied in another human being, actively affects other people's oxytocin systems if they are receptive to it? This would make those seeking help less anxious, it would lessen the pain and help to relax them. This happens not only through the physical touch but also because they mentally open up and accept help and support from the surroundings. In doing so, they activate their own oxytocin system. The effects via inner closeness amplify the effects of outer closeness.

Which people can trigger these beneficial effects? It could, of course, be anyone who is kind, and who instils confidence and trust. An important group consists of people who help others, such as doctors, nurses, clergy, teachers and mentors, in other words, individuals who help others, but also those who can provide something that the person wants. In the latter case, it might be a question of motivation and not just the need of help.

Reliance and trust towards a person can, of course, be worked on. One may ask the question whether the open channel that can arise between a psychotherapist and the patient, when reliance and trust has been created and that allows change in the patient, is partly due to the patient opening up their own oxytocin release through inner closeness, when fear and mistrust disappear. Then, the patient gets access to his or her own ability for calm, reduced stress and change, which might previously have been turned off.

Outer and inner touch is enhanced

Moreover, if the supporting and helping person touches or holds the person who is being treated, the effects are enhanced. This activates the oxytocin system from the skin as well. To be warmed, held, supported and touched, physically as well as emotionally, gives a double impact. A doctor who puts his/her hand on the patient, but who also takes the time to listen and is very kind and secure, will have much better effects than the doctor who writes out an anonymous telephone prescription or who sits and types on the computer with his/her back to the patient. Quite simply this happens because he or she triggers the patient's oxytocin system and thus the patient's own healing system in two different co-operating ways.

The placebo effect

In the medical world there is a concept known as placebo. It is a Latin word meaning 'I shall please'. This is how the placebo effect is described in the *National Encyclopaedia*: 'An effect of treatment not dependent on the specific elements of the treatment (e.g. the pharmacological active ingredient of a medicine) ... in medicine a term for something that is used as a treatment measure and deemed to not have any real biological effect on the process of the disease or of the symptoms.'

According to a now generally held theory the placebo effect in large parts depends on positive expectations resulting from the conditioning associated with previous experiences in similar situations. Such experiences could also be negative and it's then called the nocebo effect. In several cases, it has been shown that the placebo and nocebo effects are true in the sense that they are physiologically measurable. The use of placebo effects for pain, through the use of ineffective substances such as sugar pills, the injection of saline, etc., increase the body's production of endorphins, which provide pain relief in a similar way, though not to the same degree, as injected morphine.

According to the above model of explanation, the placebo effect could, above all, be linked to positive expectations and memorisation. However, there is a completely different aspect of the placebo effect and that is the effect of the person who recommends a certain type of treatment or prescribes a medicine. For example, in the assessment that a patient immediately makes about the person who is treating them, they include their medical or other competence but also their personality and approach. If the person who is treating the patient makes the patient feel calm and trusting, the patient listens and takes on board the advice and recommendations. This also activates the rest of the oxytocin system and thus reduces the patient's anxiety. He or she becomes calm and relaxed and additionally the mechanisms connected to nutritional uptake and healing are stimulated.

When the patient trusts the person who is treating them, their self-healing system is activated. If the person who is treating them has the qualities of a doula, in other words the ability to instil trust and security in the patient, then he or she has already activated the patient's own oxytocin system and thus created stress-reducing, pain-relieving and healing effects. Perhaps these effects account for the 50 per cent that the placebo effect amounts to in studies of drugs that cause pain relief. It might be worth mentioning again that oxytocin affects the pain system by increasing the activity in the endogenous endorphin system.

This may explain why it has been possible to show that endorphins are released in connection with the placebo-induced pain reduction. It also means that it is possible to activate parts of our oxytocin system and in this way create relaxation and healing without us knowing about it and without medication. Perhaps some people are particularly adept at creating trust and thereby stimulating our own calm and peace system and our self-healing system?

Today, there are intense debates about the effect of alternative or complementary therapies. In some large scientifically evaluated studies, many of these therapies proved to be more or less ineffective. Still these therapies help many people. Perhaps it is the combination of the interest in the patient and the touch, which is included in many of these treatments, that exerts the effects, since it activates the self-healing systems. Is this not what's called the art of healing?

There are also studies showing that certain antidepressants, so called SSRIs, have a much better effect if the doctor who prescribes the tablets gets to meet the patient several times. The part of the effect that is the placebo, which is mediated via the oxytocin system, is reinforced by repeated contact, since reliance and trust increase, just as oxytocin gives rise to much more long-term effects when administered frequently compared to being administered only once. It's the activity in the self-healing system that is being reinforced.

The effect of the doula or placebo is, of course, not

restricted to the people who help us with our health. It could be a teacher, priest, mentor, or any person who is conveying something to us. But if that person scares us, they fail, because then our defence system switches on. We do not listen and we don't receive. On the other hand, if he or she conveys calm and security our defence is lowered and our brain is not only open for the activation of the self-healing system but also to information and change.

8

When closeness is replaced by nutrients

When we humans lived as hunter-gatherers, it was probably not always that easy to find food. However, it was probably easier to get the need for physical closeness satisfied because of the proximity to the others in the group. Today, it seems to be the other way around. Nutrition is available in abundance, at least in our western world. You simply go to the shop and you can buy as much food as you like. Closeness, however, has become in short supply for many.

The need for hunger, food hunger, is a need that is distinguished from the need for closeness or contact with skin, known as skin hunger, which Harlow's work with rhesus monkeys clearly demonstrated. Food hunger expresses our need for nutrition and is satisfied by food. Skin hunger expresses our need for closeness and is satisfied by close contact. Food makes you full, and closeness makes you calm and secure. But you can also become calm and feel well by eating food, and therefore ingestion of food can, to a certain extent, substitute for closeness. Could there be a link between a lack of closeness and the desire for, or even craving for, food?

Food in the stomach creates calm and peace

As stated above, food doesn't just make you become full, it also creates a feeling of well-being, calmness and security. Some individuals might, therefore, compensate for a lack of closeness by eating too much. But Harlow's results with the rhesus monkeys showed that the contentment that was created by nutrition wasn't sufficient for the baby monkeys. They also needed closeness to develop into normal individuals. Therefore, to receive calm and well-being from food (or drink) must be seen as a secondary or back-up solution, opted for when closeness isn't available.

We know a lot about how our digestive system works and how the need for food is regulated. When we eat, we put food into our stomach to be further transported down to the small intestine where it is broken down into small components, which are then absorbed from the intestine and distributed in the body. To some extent, our hunger and feelings of fullness are governed by the concentration of nutrients, particularly sugar, in the bloodstream which affects the areas in the hypothalamus that deal with hunger and feelings of fullness.

But much of the information about the nutritional status takes place via nerves, just as information about the status of the skin is mediated via nerves. The presence of nutrients in the small intestine, particularly fat and protein, leads to hormones such as cholecystokinin and secretin being released from the bowel wall, and these activate the vagal nerve, which connects the gastrointestinal tract with the brain. In this way, satiety impulses from the gastrointestinal tract are conveyed to the brain.

When the vagal nerves are activated in response to a meal a feeling of fullness is created but other changes are induced. You might become calm, relaxed and even sleepy after eating, especially if you've eaten a lot of proteins and fat. But you can also experience a general feeling of well-being, and become more social and friendly. In addition, you can tolerate pain better. It hurts less at the dentist if you have food in your

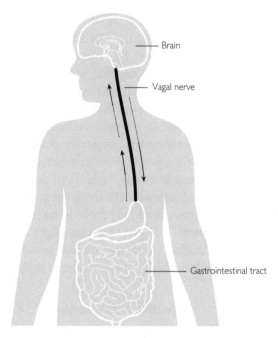

Illustration of the vagal nerve connecting the brain with the gastrointestinal tract via descending (efferent or motor) nerve fibres and via ascending (afferent or sensory) nerve fibres.

stomach than if you are hungry.

Note that these are exactly the same effects that can be triggered by touching the skin, namely, pleasure, reduced fear and increased social interaction, as well as calm and peace and relaxation. Perhaps it does not come as a surprise that the gastrointestinal hormones, which are transmitted via ascending nerve fibres in the vagal nerve, lead to the release of oxytocin in the brain. There is thus a kind of similarity between the functions in the skin and in the gastrointestinal tract – our outside and our inside. You release oxytocin, become calm, trusting and relaxed and socially interactive in response to both food intake and touch – the difference being that you also become full when you eat.

It is also interesting that the gastrointestinal tract develops in utero as an invagination of the skin. From this developmental perspective it is, therefore, perhaps not so strange that 'touching of our inside' gives rise to effects that are similar to those caused by 'touching of our outside'. It would even be possible to say that we have a kind of inner relationship with the food that we have swallowed.

Taken together, this means that the hunger for closeness and the hunger for food are partly interchangeable. If you don't have any way of managing the hunger for closeness and touch – you might not have a family or other relative or perhaps you think that touching is uncomfortable – you can always choose the inner touch and instead eat to feel good and become calm. Sandwiches and other food may replace the reassuring outer touch and closeness. It is just that you might eat more than your nutritional needs, which might result in various forms of food addictions and obesity. It is not a good solution.

Warmth is important

Most people have probably also noticed that the temperature of the food plays a part. A hot soup doesn't just make you full but it makes you feel warm and comfortable inside during the winter whereas a cold drink would have completely the opposite effect. Young children who have drunk warm milk in the evening quickly become calm and fall asleep easily. If the milk was cold, they would not relax as quickly.

The skin also likes warmth. A nice, warm bath makes us relax and many people feel very good when they are 'sunbathing'. They become happier, more satisfied and more communicative by being in the warm and touching sun. The nice feeling that the sun's rays can bestow is reflected not least in the faces of the people sitting outside on the stairs of the Royal Dramatic Theatre in Stockholm and receiving the first sunbeams of spring! In this context, we can also remind ourselves of the newborn baby lying against its mother after birth, becoming more and more relaxed in response to the mother's warmth.

Food in the stomach creates trust

When we eat with other people we tend to judge them as familiar and harmless, and we think that they are friendly and that we can trust them. This increased trust is also a sign that oxytocin has been released as the administration of oxytocin creates trust.

Consider how a businessman behaves when he's about to sign a contract. He treats the client to a nice meal, perhaps with a glass of wine or two. He knows from experience that there is a much better chance that the deal will be made if they eat together. Everyone feels good and becomes calm, and trust is increased in all parties, thus improving the chances for a signed contract or some form of agreement. This effect can be explained in purely physiological terms, starting with the presence of food in the gastrointestinal tract, which, via a release of the hormone cholecystokinin, activates the vagal nerves which in turn activate the release of oxytocin in the brain – and through this trust is achieved. The oxytocin that is subsequently released in the brain induces trust but also creates a feeling of calm and relaxation, and enhances social skills.

Even deeper bonds and relationships can be reinforced with food. It is said, for example, that the way to a man's heart is through his stomach. Your mother's meatballs contain more than meat! In the U.S. there are also special techniques that use food as a way of reaching young people who distrust the community. These individuals have often had a very difficult childhood and these young people don't trust their fellow humans and therefore don't care about what they say. Sometimes, therapists can reach these youths if they share a meal with them in a safe environment. Because food and nutrition can increase trust, you can get them to open up and in this way become susceptible to new information, which could lead to them being able to change their life situation.

We don't know much about what happens in the gastrointestinal tract in humans who are exposed to situations that lead to their reliance on the world around them being disturbed. But one can assume that the digestion and nutrient intake might be impaired. If you shut yourself off from other people, in other words if you refrain from closeness and touch, perhaps the function in the gastrointestinal tract follows suit since the mechanisms that regulate closeness and nutrient intake are so intimately linked.

Many people who are grieving and feel abandoned lose their appetite – as if they close the gate to the stomach when they've lost an important link to someone they love. Others compensate by excessive eating and drinking.

With food in the stomach, we become more generous

Those who do not get enough food have nothing to give. A person who is starving becomes more selfish. When it comes to life and survival, consideration for other people disappears. The hungry take whatever food they can lay their hands on, even if this has an impact on their fellow humans. This effect was seen in particular in the concentration camps during World War II. Without food, there is no morality or, as the German writer Bertolt Brecht expressed it, 'Erst kommt das Fressen, dann kommt die Moral' (first comes the feeding, then comes morality).

If we turn this around, it means that if you're full up, you're also more generous. Shakespeare touched on this when he let Julius Caesar say that he wanted to have round and nice people around him. He could also have said that he wanted people around him that eat well.

There is an interesting animal model that shows how important the gastrointestinal tract is for us to be generous. In these experiments, the researchers cut the vagal nerve, the nerve that connects the gastrointestinal tract and the brain, in a group of female rats that were feeding their young. Despite this, the pups continued to feed from their mothers and the mothers continued to eat as normal. However, after a few days

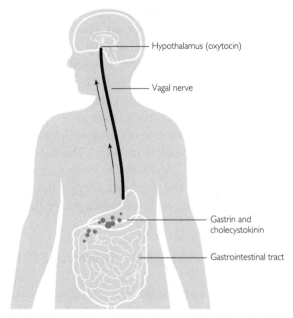

When the stomach and intestine contain nutrients (mainly fats and proteins) the hormone cholecystokinin is released in the upper small intestine. This results in the upward vagal fibres being activated, which results in oxytocin release, as illustrated by the arrows.

the mothers stopped producing milk and were less caring of their young. It was found that the pups' suckling no longer resulted in oxytocin release, which explained why the mothers no longer produced any milk or took care of their pups. Instead, the mother became fatter!

Why would this happen? Well, normally the information that there is food in the gastrointestinal tract is transmitted via the vagal nerve to the brain. When this signal was absent in the rats whose vagal nerve was cut the rats' brains 'thought' that they had not received any food and therefore no oxytocin was released. The rat mothers stopped giving milk to their pups. Instead the rat mothers retained and stored up the calories in their bodies. An altruistic behaviour turned into a selfish behaviour.

You can actually induce both maternal behaviour and milk ejection in female rats that are feeding their pups by administering the fullness hormone CCK – yet a further demonstration of the strong link between feeling full and generosity on both a nutritional and a behavioural level. In this sense the gastrointestinal satiety hormone CCK becomes the mother of the mother hormone oxytocin.

The way that oxytocin is associated with generosity can also be seen in breastfeeding mothers. The more oxytocin that is released during a breastfeed the more milk the mother produces for her child and the more socially interactive she becomes according to the well established personality profiles.

Touch improves the gastrointestinal function

Many of you will have heard the stories of the children who were raised in an orphanage and died, despite having adequate food and hygienic care. The exception was the child who slept by the door in the dormitory, which each night was lifted up and cared for by the night staff. This story shows that nutrition and hygiene are not enough and that touch and closeness are essential for our survival. One of the reasons why the children in the orphanage did not survive was that they couldn't use the food that they were given for growth. This is partly due to the fact that, in the absence of touch, the hormones in the gastrointestinal tract that take care of digestion and nutrient absorption are not released in sufficient quantities. Touch increases the activity in some branches of the outward-reaching vagal nerve, which helps the food in the gastrointestinal tract to release digestive hormones, thereby optimising the digestive capacity and the use of the ingested nutrients for growth purposes.

When a newborn baby has skin-to-skin contact with its mother, the level of certain gastrointestinal hormones such as gastrin and cholecystokinin decreases. These hormones are of importance for digestion, the assimilation of nutrients and for growth. In contrast, the hormone levels rise more in these infants when the food finally arrives in the digestive tract than in infants who are not in skin-to-skin contact. It is clear, therefore, that digestion is more effective when it is accompanied by skin-to-skin contact. Both the reduction in hormone levels before breastfeeding and the enhanced rise after the breastfeed are due to the fact that skin contact, via the touch nerves, increases the activity in the vagal nerve. Both of these effects are facilitated by oxytocin released in the brain.

Another way to increase the activity in the vagal nerve is to let young children suckle properly by breastfeeding or by sucking on a dummy while being tube fed. The suckling, which is a much more powerful type of stimulation compared to touch, activates additional nerve fibres in the outward-reaching vagal nerve and the release of gastrointestinal hormones is enhanced. The oxytocin nerves in the brain are part of the chain of nerves which contribute towards the increase in activity in the vagal nerve in connection with touch and suckling and the consequent stimulation of the release of gastrointestinal hormones.

Gastrointestinal hormones are also released in response to suckling in breastfeeding mothers. In this way the mother's digestion and ability to store and use nutrients for milk production are enhanced.

Gastrointestinal tract and love

If you measure the levels of gastrin (a hormone that is produced in the stomach and stimulates the secretion of gastric juice) in mothers a few days after giving birth, it is found that mothers who have had a lot of skin-to-skin contact with their baby immediately after birth have lower gastrin levels compared to the mothers who have had less skin-to-skin contact. Obviously the reduction of gastrin levels which is created by skin-to-skin contact in mothers after birth has become permanent.

The mother's gastrin levels also reflect the degree of

bonding with the child. The lower the gastrin levels, the greater is her sense of closeness to her baby. Since the bond between mother and child is initiated by oxytocin, and because the oxytocin levels in the mother have been shown to be related to the level of bonding to the child as well as to calm and positive feelings, it is most likely that the gastrin level is a consequence of oxytocin release in the brain. This relationship is also supported by studies showing a reduction in gastrin levels in rats after the administration of oxytocin.

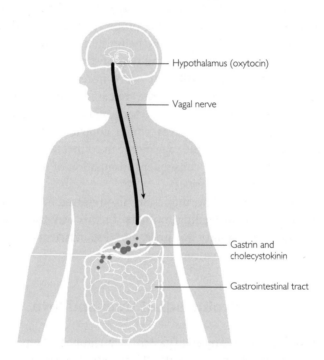

Oxytocin nerves from the hypothalamus can, via the effects in the brainstem where the function of the vagal nerve is controlled via the downward-reaching vagal fibres, affect some aspects of gastrointestinal function, such as the release of the hormones gastrin and cholecystokinin in the gastrointestinal tract.

Homesickness can take the form
of an expression of hunger

It is not uncommon for homesickness, which in reality is a longing for closeness to those who you are close to and the familiar home environment, to manifest itself in an increase in hunger after a period of decreased appetite. This is something that many young people who have left home have experienced. It is not unusual for them, in this situation, to eat too much and this can lead to weight problems and eating disorders that might be difficult to balance.

There are studies that show that the functions of the gastrointestinal tract, namely the production of gastric juices and substances that break down food, also increase with homesickness when the stomach is empty. In an American study, young men who were called in for military service were studied. It was discovered that those who were homesick were more at risk of developing gastric ulcers. This is understandable since ulcers are to a certain extent caused by excess formation of gastric juices and enzymes for breaking down the food. Digestion is not only activated when you are hungry and long for food, but also in some individuals when they are separated from and long for those that they like and depend on.

It is probable that the level of gastrin during homesickness increases and this in turn results in an increase in the production of gastric juices and elevated levels of the enzymes that are necessary to break down the food. Consequently the stomach lining becomes irritated and this can be experienced as a kind of craving or hunger that can only be subdued by food. Perhaps *Heliobacter pylori*, the bacterium that contributes to ulcer formation, thrives and grows when the empty stomach contains gastric juice. Since gastrin is a hormone that stimulates gastric acid secretion it's not appropriate to have high gastrin levels when the stomach is empty. Viewed from this angle, it is even more interesting that touch and closeness lower the gastrin levels.

When you are at home, you have access to closeness and touch from your loved ones. This has the effect of lowering the gastrin level and thus gastric juice production, thereby protecting the digestive tract. The link to touch is further demonstrated by studies showing a similar reduction of gastrin levels during massage and touch in both animals and humans. Other studies show that people with low gastrin levels have low levels of anxiety and have a high social competence.

The reverse also applies because high levels of gastrin have been associated with worry and anxiety. If you administer a type of gastrin to humans called pentagastrin, which passes into the brain, they can suffer panic attacks and anxiety. Individuals with high gastrin levels have been shown to be at an increased risk of worrying and of developing myocardial infarction.

Collectively, all of these studies show that it is favourable to have low gastrin levels between meals and that they are kept low by touch and closeness. Oxytocin levels in the brain, and also bonding and trust, are linked to low gastrin levels and, as described above, touch and closeness may release oxytocin.

These results further support the close relationship between oxytocin levels in the brain, the levels of hormones in the gastrointestinal tract and its ability to function well. Or in other words, the gastrointestinal tract's function is improved by close relationships and you could perhaps even use the levels of gastrointestinal hormones as a measure of closeness and happiness! Love and good relationships are reflected in the levels of gastrointestinal tract hormones and gastrointestinal function!

9

Closeness provides good health and a longer life

Most of us know that children who do not get closeness and touch do not fare well and that children who do not receive love fail to grow as expected and that, in extreme cases, they might even die. On the other hand, as we described earlier, touch and closeness between a child and its parents increases growth and development such as in premature infants.

There are a few mammals that live in life-long 'marriages'. These include some types of vole, some monkeys and the *Tupaia*, which is a kind of tree shrew. When these animals mate, they are bonded to one another for life. When one of them dies, the partner dies soon after. The fellowship and being together are, therefore, essential for living for these couple-making animals. A similar phenomenon is sometimes seen in humans, and two very close individuals will pass away in quick succession. It is as if their togetherness has kept the flame of life alight.

There are several studies showing that stable and good relationships are also good for the health of adults. The risk of developing certain types of illnesses, including depression, anxiety disorders and cardiovascular disease, is lower for people who live in pairs. People who live in happy relationships and who have a good sex life even look younger than other men and women of the same age. However, these correlations seem to apply more to men than women. It could, therefore be slightly dangerous for a man to live on his own. Many men seem to sense this and after a separation soon begin a new relationship. Women, on the other hand, appear to manage better without a special partner compared to men. Perhaps this is because women often have multiple close relationships, such as with their parents, children and friends.

For women it is, of course, also important for their health to live in a couple relationship, but it has been shown that this is only beneficial if the relationship is good. The Swedish researcher Kristina Orth-Gomér has shown that women who feel unsafe and scared in their relationships are at an increased risk of developing cardiovascular disease. This means that it is not only the existence of a relationship per se that is important but also its quality.

How can positive relationships improve health?

We will now go back to the book's beginning and remind ourselves of what happens in the relationship between the parent and the newborn child. We can conclude that skin-to-skin contact makes both adults and children more social and they feel better. The activity in the sympathetic nervous system is subdued so that the blood pressure is lowered and the concentration of the stress hormone cortisol is lowered because the activity in the HPA-axis is reduced. At the same time, digestion, nutritional storage and the systems that are involved in healing and growth are all improved due to the increase of activity in the vagal/parasympathetic nervous system. In this way, both body and brain are affected and all these effects are obviously good for the health. It is healthy to tone down the activity in the systems connected with tension and stress and to stimulate activity in the systems that deal with restorative and healing processes. All these effects are associated with the release of oxytocin which is created by closeness between parent and child.

Stress-related illness is counteracted by close relationships

Cardiovascular diseases are often related to stress and an elevated activity in the sympathetic nervous system. The illness-reducing effects which are associated with close relationships can thus be due to the fact that the stress levels are reduced, but can obviously also be connected to the increased activity in the systems that deal with healing. With this in mind, it becomes quite logical that close relationships are good for the health since intimacy promotes the release of oxytocin.

We have already described how oxytocin can suppress not only the activity in the HPA axis, and therefore lower levels of cortisol, but also the activity of the cardiovascular system, which leads to the lowering of blood pressure and a slower heart rate. Recently, it has also been shown that inflammation in the vessel walls, which is considered to contribute towards atherosclerosis, is also counteracted by oxytocin.

Nutritional uptake, growth and healing also benefit from oxytocin. This happens on many levels so that, for example, the activities in the gastrointestinal tract and the parasympathetic nervous system are enhanced. This also means that the individual who is continuously exposed to oxytocin not only becomes less stressed but also the ability for recovery and repair is amplified. These effects may be one of the reasons why close relationships are linked to good health.

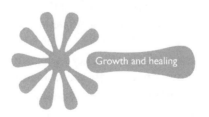

Growth and healing

In parallel with oxytocin's ability to suppress the activity of the sympathetic nervous system and increase the activity of the parasympathetic nervous system in the body, the systems in the brain, which are connected to wakefulness, stress and aggression, and growth, learning and memory respectively, are affected in an analogous manner.

As stated before, the effects of closeness – that is touch, warmth and light pressure – depend on the activation of sensory nerves which lead to the reactions described above and the release of oxytocin. These closeness reactions, which obviously also include positive signals from other senses, are repeated to different degrees throughout life during each single positive meeting between individuals.

Over time, the short-term effects that are triggered during each single meeting will turn into the chronic changes which were described earlier. By then, oxytocin has affected the activities in other signalling systems in a long-term way. As an example, a few injections of oxytocin can lower the blood pressure and level of stress hormones in a rat for several weeks after the oxytocin was administered. Also, as we have seen, a woman who has given birth several times is protected against stress-related diseases (for example high blood pressure and type 2 diabetes) because of her exposure to the effects of oxytocin over a long period of her life. It is exactly the same mechanism that makes good relationships protect against illnesses because the direct closeness to people that we like and feel safe with continuously triggers oxytocin release and its associated reactions.

We humans can obviously also react positively to meetings with other people without touching them directly. It is as if the very fact that we like, trust and have faith in another person is enough to initiate the oxytocin-mediated effect pattern.

It is as if 'inner touch', or the feeling and experience of warmth and love, creates the same psychological effects as direct touch and warmth do through physiological mechanisms. There are also studies showing that blood pressure is lower in individuals who are involved in good relationships and that blood pressure is connected to levels of oxytocin – the higher the oxytocin levels, the lower the levels of oxytocin.

Early closeness and health as an adult

Extra touch or the administration of oxytocin to newborns can create life-long effects. We have earlier described how touch, warmth and closeness after birth produce rats that are more social and calmer and that they have decreased stress-levels and lower blood pressure compared to those that haven't had the extra stimulation. If you administer oxytocin to newborn pups, the adult rats get a decrease in blood pressure, become calmer and more pain-resistant. In addition they grow faster. These results support the assumption that oxytocin affects the individual early in life and that these effects can become permanent. The effects are life-long because newborns are more easily influenced than adults and are open to different kinds of imprinting or learning or even epigenetic influences. The reduced fear and the increased social capacity of the rats that receive a lot of closeness and touch as newborns have been linked to an increased activity of oxytocin in the adult animal's brain, particularly in the amygdala, an area which is of importance for the regulation of social interaction and the levels of fear or anxiety. This suggests that the rat mothers stimulate the release of oxytocin in the pups when they lick them. The American researcher Neil Schneiderman from Miami in Florida and his co-workers have shown how touch and the administration of oxytocin to baby rabbits can prevent the development of atherosclerosis in adult rabbits.

Their experiments have shown that rabbits who have a diet rich in fat as babies develop hardening of the artery walls when they become adults whereas this does not happen in the same way in rabbits who receive a normal diet. But if the baby rabbits that receive the diet rich in fat also get extra touch, the vascular changes do not occur later in life. The same beneficial effects are obtained if the baby rabbits receive extra oxytocin when they are young. The results thus show that touching of the young rabbits results in the release of endogenous oxytocin which then protects against atherosclerosis.

It is not yet known if human children who have had access to extra closeness when young develop a certain resistance to stress-related illnesses when they are adults in a similar way. However, it is likely that this is the case since we know from studies of their behaviour when they are around one year old that that they are more responsive to social cues and that they can handle stress better if they receive closeness immediately after birth. Furthermore, it has been shown that the opposite is true. Children who have been exposed to stress during pregnancy have been shown to have an increased risk of developing high blood pressure, certain cardiovascular diseases and diabetes. Children who have been victims of many separations early on in life have an increased risk of anxiety and depression as adults. You might, of course just as well turn the argument on its head and say that the absence of stress early on in life protects against these types of illnesses! This is, however, not the whole truth since it seems as if a rich supply of closeness in early life takes the development one step further. The individuals become more socially interactive, calmer and more relaxed. In other words, the calm and connection system becomes more strongly expressed.

It is, as we have seen, not just the child who benefits from closeness during the first few weeks after birth. The calming effects in the mother can last for a very long time and can even protect her in the long term from certain stress-related illnesses later in life. As mentioned earlier, clinical investigations have shown that women who breastfeed are 'dose dependently' protected from getting certain cardiovascular diseases such as myocardial infarction, stroke and hypertension. They are also to some extent protected against type 2 diabetes – the type of diabetes that occurs in adults or older people. This protection against certain stress-related illnesses that has been observed in women who breastfeed is likely to be due to the repeated oxytocin release that takes place during lactation. The most important conclusion is that closeness and good relationships continue to affect our health in a positive way throughout our life, even if the effects are stronger if closeness is applied early in life.

Man's best friend makes its masters healthy

A relationship that is important to many, and which has also been shown to be important to health, is that of a beloved pet. The dog is related to the wolf. Dogs have been bred for many purposes and based on many characteristics and abilities. By choosing to breed the animals that were unafraid of humans, we eventually arrived at today's companion dogs. During the time of breeding for tameness, the dog's appearance changed, the ears started to droop and the tail could bend upwards. The fur changed colour and could even be spotty. Probably the faces changed too and became more 'baby-like'. Perhaps it is the combination of the changed appearance and the friendliness that dogs show us humans that makes us like them so much? Perhaps selective breeding for these traits resulted in an enhanced oxytocin system in domesticated dogs, thus creating the tame and friendly dogs who have become man's best friend? Is this why we are not afraid of companion dogs and often want to approach them without even knowing them? There is no doubt that most pet dogs are very fond of being stroked and hugged, something that adult wolves most probably wouldn't like.

There are countless examples of how dogs and humans can 'tune in' to each other and become very close. The so-called alert dogs are an example of dogs which are of great help to humans. These dogs are trained to recognise when their master's blood sugars are too low or when an epileptic seizure is on its way. In the first instance, the dog retrieves a small bag of sugar and sweets so that the threatening attack of low blood sugar can be stopped and in the second case, the dog immediately makes sure that other people are alerted who can then assist during an epileptic seizure. It is amazing what these dogs can do.

Anyone with a dog is often healthy

There is today an overwhelming amount of literature that shows that those who have dogs are generally healthier than those who do not have dogs. In particular, dog owners are protected against stress of various kinds. It has also been demonstrated that dog owners have a better prognosis if they have had a heart attack compared to those who don't have a dog. They also have lower blood pressure.

Of course, you think, this must be because dog owners who are out walking their dogs are more physically fit, something that tends to lead to better health. And it is certainly part of the truth. But even in studies that take into account the physical activity it has been shown that dog owners have a lower stress level and a reduced risk of developing certain heart problems. It is, therefore, something more than simply exercise that affects the dog owners positively. Many studies show that it is also good for social competence to have an animal, especially a dog. For children, it can be very important and positive. Those who have had a dog as a child will benefit from it even as an adult.

The beneficial effects on health and on the ability for social interaction are probably due to dogs and dog owners touching each other and liking each other. The owner strokes and hugs the dog. When they know each other well, the mere presence of the dog will be calming. When the dog and owner have bonded, they also affect each other positively through the invisible tie the bonding brings. The dog affects its owners both through physical and mental closeness.

We have seen how the oxytocin effects are made permanent and become prolonged after repeated administrations. Since the owners have their dog close by most of the time, they receive small regular doses of oxytocin and therefore develop a more chronic activation of the calm and connection system.

It is most likely these more chronic effects of the oxytocin that give rise to the health-promoting effects.

What about other animals? Curiously enough, it has not been possible to show any de-stressing and health-promoting effects from having a cat. Perhaps this is because a cat doesn't always enter an equally close relationship with humans as the dog but rather lives a bit more distantly? But it may actually simply be because cat owners haven't been studied as well as dog owners and therefore the potential positive impacts might have been missed.

Animals in the healthcare system

In many places, animals are used in the healthcare system because of their beneficial effects on humans. Cats and dogs spread joy and happiness around them and can motivate older people to exercise more and generally become more active. Both cats and dogs are very much appreciated, for example, in homes for the elderly and the mentally ill. It is even possible that visits by dogs could replace some drug treatment in nursing homes since dogs also seem to create joy and reduce aggression in the elderly, especially if they are suffering from dementia. But this remains to be shown. Should this be the case, it might even be profitable to use dogs in the healthcare system.

In some places, dogs are also used as therapists, especially when treating children. Sometimes the presence of a dog can solve difficult situations and relationships. It's as if it is much easier to talk about difficult things with a dog or if a dog is present. This is partly because the dog is quiet and loyal, and it never gossips, but dogs also seem to increase the ability in some people to express difficult things both individually and together with other people. Dogs have a very calming effect and it has been shown that children can concentrate better on their homework if they have a dog in the room. All these effects could be linked to a release of oxytocin in humans in response to the different types of encounters with the dogs.

EVEN COWS AND OTHER ANIMALS

In many places, farm animals are used to help people back to recuperate and return to good health. Being on a farm and helping with the animals also creates opportunities for closeness and for the possibility to experience a certain kind of relationship. In many parts of Europe, it is common to let tired, depressed and anxious people spend time with animals in an agricultural environment. In Norway, Bente Berget and Bjarne Braastad have shown that the mentally ill felt better and became calmer if they were able to spend a few afternoons a week together with animals on a farm.

As we described in the chapter about the mammalian heritage, it seems as though cows, who naturally have high levels of oxytocin when they are being milked or giving birth, have a calming effect on the other cows in the barn. There are also many stories about people who grew up on a dairy farm having experienced how the cows also had a calming effect on the humans. It has been said that if babies with colic are taken out to the most peaceful cow in the barn the colic pains stop and the babies become calmer. Perhaps the oxytocin-packed cows that were regularly milked released a fragrance that also had an effect on us humans? Perhaps the airborne information was more important for ancient humans than it is for today's highly educated individuals? Or is it that we humans are still affected by pheromones to a higher degree than we think, but we don't know about it?

The dog and the human react in the same way

This book is written from a human's perspective and therefore we have stressed the importance of closeness between humans and dogs, especially from the perspective of the owners. But it is of course equally important for animals such as dogs to feel good. And why wouldn't it be like that? The type of interaction which involves close contact, physically and mentally, works in both directions. The fact is that not only dogs but also cows can become calmer by being stroked and touched by humans that they know or are not afraid of. They react exactly like us by decreasing their pulse rate and blood pressure, as well as by a decrease in their levels of the stress hormone cortisol. In dogs the level of oxytocin simultaneously rises! What happens in other animal species is not yet known.

This means that dogs and many other animals might also benefit from closeness and touch not only from their own species but also from us humans. At this level, all mammals are the same.

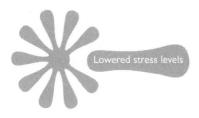

Lowered stress levels

Oxytocin and massage

At the beginning of life, closeness and touch are vitally important, but the need for closeness remains throughout life. And of course, most people receive touch and closeness from their nearest and dearest. But perhaps a small deficit in the 'touch account' has arisen in our individualistic and hectic world where many people live alone. One sign of this latent lack of touch is that people are seeking ways to compensate for this loss or absence. The high demands for various forms of massage or touch therapies at the present time are an expression of this need. People have simply discovered that different types of touch and massage make them feel good.

Today there are a large number of scientific studies showing that massage has many beneficial effects. Professor Tiffany Field at the Touch Research Institute in Miami has made pioneering contributions to document its effects. She started by showing that premature babies grow more quickly if they receive massage and that they can leave the hospital after a shorter time. She has since performed a variety of studies in old and young, men and women, as well as on healthy people and individuals with various illnesses. In conclusion, her research results show that massage reduces anxiety, stress and depression. Massage also increases well-being, improves concentration and learning, and enhances social interaction.

There are many types of massage and touch therapies. In the classic massage, the muscles are mainly massaged while the skin is the focus of treatment in touch therapies. The touch therapies (for example, tactile stimulation, touch or light massage) may include stroking of the whole body or, as in the Rosen method (a technique developed by the physiotherapist Marion Rosen), a more localised light touch designed to induce relaxation, especially in the muscles that affect breathing.

The different treatments do not produce exactly the same effects in everyone. The effects depend partly on the type of treatment that is provided. Often, the effects are most evident when there is something missing or out of sorts. The effects that are created by massage and touch are also due to the specific needs that the people who are being treated may have. For some, it is important to receive a hard kneading of the muscles to get them to relax and to kickstart the blood circulation. These people naturally detect the effects mostly on the muscles but have probably also experienced an increased calm and well-being as a result of the treatment.

Others, and perhaps especially the elderly, often suffer from lack of touch and for them it is more important to experience soft stimulation of the skin. There are many studies showing that old people feel good when they receive various forms of touch therapies. They become calmer, and sleep better. Their relationship with the staff improves and they generally have a better quality of life. During infant massage the aim is, above all, to increase the contact between the parents and the child and to create calm and harmony in the child.

For touch to be perceived as pleasant and to give rise to positive effects, it is also required that you are touched by someone that you know and like or by someone that you accept for other reasons. It is also become increasingly apparent that the approach of the person offering the treatment is of great importance. It is essential that the therapist treats the patient in a respectful manner. A treatment must be given with soft warm hands and the person offering the treatment must be mentally present and have good intentions. There is a big difference between being touched by a soft and warm hand or a cold and hard hand. With cold and hard hands and an absent and uninterested mind, the positive results are absent and in the worst case scenario could turn into a stress reaction. The latter can be experienced as very uncomfortable and unpleasant.

Not everyone likes touch

There is also a large group of people who on the whole do not like touch. Some of them have previously had unpleasant experiences that can be connected to touch. For these individuals those unpleasant forgotten memories might surface in connection with touch and, in these situations, stress and defence reactions are triggered instead of calm and relaxation. Such reactions occur on an instinctive level and can be very difficult to overcome.

Other people seem to have a congenital inability to tolerate touch and can, regardless of previous experiences, think that touch feels uncomfortable – as if it grinds and stings. For them, it may even be difficult to wear certain types of clothes because the fabric irritates. Perhaps it is due to some kind of 'incorrect wiring' between the various touch and pain nerves? It is also not uncommon that individuals with autistic traits, that is individuals who have difficulties with social contacts with others, also have problems with touch. Perhaps these characteristics are connected?

Results from studies of massage and touch

Below are results from a range of studies in which various forms of massage or touch have been used and where the purpose of the treatment and the observed treatment results have been very different.

CALMER AT KINDERGARTEN

In a study carried out in day-care centres, led by Professor Anne-Liis von Knorring at the Department of Neuroscience at Uppsala University Hospital, researchers examined how massage affected the children's behaviour. Preliminary observations had found that children who receive massage became calmer and functioned better socially. In the study, massage was provided during a ten-minute period during the rest-time in the middle of the day by a member of staff. The massage was provided according to a particular schedule and all staff who participated in the study had been trained to use the same massage technique that had been used at Axelsson's Gymnastic Institute in Stockholm. Of course, the children decided themselves if they wanted to partake in the study. To be able to evaluate the effects of the massage, the children in departments where massage had yet to be introduced were also studied. Both the staff and the parents helped to evaluate the effectiveness of the massage therapy.

When the results were evaluated, at first there seemed to be no difference between the children who had received massage and the ones who hadn't. However, if the choice was made to study the most active and unsettled children in both groups, a difference could be detected six months later. At that time, the children who had received massage had become calmer compared to those in the control group. The massage-dependent effects were prolonged and had even improved after twelve months. What was most noticeable was that the treatment with massage had suppressed aggressive behaviour in the boys who were extremely unsettled. At the same time, their ability to function in a social context had improved and they also had less pain. The parents and the staff were unanimous in their assessments. The positive effects spread through the departments. The groups of children functioned better and the staff's well-being increased. Doesn't this sound familiar? Decreased aggression and increased social interaction are typical manifestations of increased oxytocin effect.

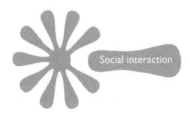

DEVELOPMENT AND CHANGE

In another study, tactile touch was given to a group of young women with problematic lives at a treatment clinic in Linköping in Sweden. These women were adults but generally had no jobs. They had been receiving counselling from qualified psychologists and sociologists for years and thus their lives were more or less functional.

Some of these women received ten treatments of tactile stimulations over a number of weeks from a trained touch therapist in addition to the counselling which continued as normal. It turned out that the women who received a 'touch-supplement' were changed in a positive way. They all felt better and their self-esteem increased. They frequently altered their static way of living. Some of them applied for jobs and others cared about their appearance in a completely different way than before. They simply became more outgoing.

The most interesting finding was that the positive changes didn't stop when the touch treatments ended, but the women who received this therapy continued to feel good for a very long time afterwards. Many of them had on their own initiative started some other form of touch therapy. They didn't just feel better; they became more active and more curious about the outside world.

BETTER COMMUNICATION
BETWEEN CHILDREN AND CAREGIVERS

In another study on children with multiple disabilities, the effect of tactile stimulation was studied. This particular treatment technique includes, in addition to touch by the hands, a 'touching approach' by the therapist, which is to be friendly and respectful.

The children lived on wards or stayed in day-care specifically for children with multiple disabilities at Bräcke Diakoni in Gothenburg, and they received ten treatments from their personal assistants. These often severely disabled children liked the treatments, and they relaxed and enjoyed themselves when the treatment was given. But perhaps the most obvious consequences of the treatment were that the relationships with the personal assistants became so much better. The disabled children could not speak but communicated in other ways. After they had received the extra touch their communication increased in many ways. They smiled more and had more eye contact with their assistants and tried to pass on what they thought and felt by the means they had available to them. Some of the children tried to give massage back. Many of the children also took more social initiatives at home with their parents or at school.

The effects were, however, not one sided. The staff also commented that their relationship with the children had deepened and become much more loving. The effect was so powerful that it spread to the other staff on the same ward where the children lived or spent time and everyone perceived work and co-operation more positively. The positive effect on the working atmosphere can also be seen as an oxytocin effect on a group level.

Again, we sense that the oxytocin release which is created

by touch, both in the receiver and the provider, may have contributed towards the increased ability and desire to communicate and to a more loving connection between them. The effects that were obtained are similar to the bonding that is created between parent and child if they have the opportunity for extra closeness early on in life.

The Rosen Method

The Rosen Method is a touch therapy developed by the physiotherapist Marion Rosen. Marion Rosen was born in Germany but moved to Sweden before the Second World War where she studied to become a physiotherapist. She was then for a long time a resident of Berkeley in the U.S. Marion Rosen says that the body remembers much more than what we humans are aware of and that small contractions in certain muscles may be linked to repressed memories of traumatic experiences. The Rosen therapist works by using a very light touch to get muscles to relax, including those that restrict breathing. While this is occurring, the patient might become aware of events that he or she has previously experienced but has repressed. When the memories become conscious, they can be handled in a better way and a blocked development can proceed. The Rosen Method is thus primarily focused on psychological development.

The Swedish Rosen therapist Annika Minnbergh and her colleagues are using the Rosen Method in war-torn Bosnia. They provide courses in the Rosen Method and treat people who have experienced traumatic events during the war. Through the warming touch and through the therapist's supporting and holding approach and the relaxation that follows the treatment, those who receive treatment get access to the memories of their horrible experiences. But they get them in a warm and safe environment and thereby they can transform the memories and discharge them. What is most amazing is that the treatment not only has a positive effect at the individual level but also allows for reconciliation between people of different races and religions. Because the war-affected individuals are no longer controlled by the terrible memories and perceived wrongs, the fear is released together with the desire for revenge. They are able to move on without really thinking about it and create new social connections within and outside of their ethnic groups and religions. When fear and aggression are released and you begin to trust in each other, life together can continue. This becomes particularly clear if the individuals who treat each other are of a different ethnicity and religion, in other words former enemies. When the Rosen Method is used in this context, it is mainly the ability of touch to release blocked memories and facilitate the re-orientation as well as the calm and peace-making effects of oxytocin which are expressed.

If the studies that are currently under way to document the effects of the Rosen Method give rise to positive results it will mean that it, and possibly other touch therapies, can become an important tool for solving problems and conflicts between people, if used with good judgement, understanding and care.

How does massage and touch work?

The fact that, in spite of great differences, we can have similar effects from various types of massage and touch therapies is because it is the hands that are the common tool. Irrespective of whether it is a strong classical massage of the muscles, a pure touch therapy or a very soft muscle-relaxing Rosen treatment, the warmth and touch mediated by the hands are part of the treatment. In turn, the touch and warmth activate the oxytocin system, particularly in the brain. At this point, just as during the closeness between parent and child, social interaction and calm are stimulated while stress reactions decrease.

There are scientific studies in which it has been shown that oxytocin levels rise in the short term in the blood of people who received massage. On the other hand, it is not that easy to measure the oxytocin levels in the human brain where the massage-related effects are exerted. But the fact that oxytocin is released into the blood as a result of massage, and that a typical oxytocin effect pattern is induced, supports oxytocin's role as an important co-ordinator of the effects of massage and other touch therapies.

Touch is part of many other alternative or complementary medical treatments as well. There is today a very inflamed debate about whether these treatments work or not. If you read the book *Trick or Treatment* by Simon Singh and Edzard Ernst, you can easily get the impression that everything except massage is a bluff. The reasons why the authors express themselves so strongly is because they claim that no scientific studies have been able to show that acupuncture or homeopathy are any more effective than control treatments.

The initial explanatory models that were used to account for the effects of these alternative or complementary treatments were rejected as impossible and improbable. That may be the case, but all patients, whether they are actively treated or part of a control group, are in close contact with the therapist. They will be thoroughly questioned about their problems and lifestyles at the first meeting and their concerns are taken seriously. Often a number of treatments are included in the different therapies and, therefore, the people who are being treated get to meet with their therapist repeatedly.

As far as acupuncture is concerned there is a substantial element of skin contact when the therapist places the needles which, when they are inserted, continue to 'touch'. New scientifically controlled studies show that treatment with a lighter kind of acupuncture needle that doesn't go as deeply into the skin gives rise to as good an effect as the needles which are inserted more deeply. This suggests that it is the skin contact, in other words touch from the therapist and from the needles, that creates the effects.

In addition, acupuncturists, osteopaths and chiropractors, and other practitioners of alternative treatments, can most certainly create many strong and positive effects that are specific to the different treatments and that may be difficult to capture in scientific studies, but they all have one feature in common which is that the touch of the skin is an important component. It would be possible to reverse the argument and say that it is impossible not to trigger the touch effects during manual therapies. This means that it is not just massage and touch but also all these other forms of therapies that, to some extent, give rise to touch-induced oxytocin effects, that is, a reduction of stress, reduction of pain and the stimulation of healing mechanisms in the body. In addition, if the therapists have the trust of their patients they can reach in via the 'trust channel' which also contributes to the release of oxytocin and therefore the healing properties.

10

The oxytocin heritage

We humans are the most developed of all the animals in the mammalian group in the sense that we have a much more developed cerebral cortex compared to other mammals. Thanks to our frontal lobes, we can plan, associate and create an existence that seems thoroughly conscious. In other mammals, it's not only the bodily processes that are governed primarily by unconscious processes that are located in the older parts of the brain, but also behaviour and various forms of relationships.

An important message of this book is that human relationships also contain components that can be attributed to our mammalian heritage. Infatuation and love create happiness and can bind together with enormous forces, not to mention jealousy with its hurt and all that it brings with the need to control and perhaps also revenge. These aspects of our relationships cannot be controlled at will; we might possibly to some extent learn to handle them.

Another important and not much considered aspect to be taken into account is that the mechanisms that create and perpetuate human relationships are a legacy of our mammalian heritage. There are many types of relationships that involve two individuals, such as the parent and the infant or the couple in love, while others comprise a number of individuals, such as family relationships or workplace relationships. Despite all the differences, there are some commonalities between these different types of relationship.

For a relationship to occur, you need in some way to get closer to the other individual and to do this you need to not be afraid of that person. You must then learn to recognise the other person. During closeness in various kinds of relationships, the body's reward system is activated and stress and tension are decreased. After some time, these reactions are automatically linked together with the other person and this makes it sufficient for the mere presence of him or her for the positive reactions to be triggered. The recognition can be through smell, hearing or sight, the latter being the most common one in humans. But the positive effects don't last indefinitely, and will subside if the members of the relationship are separated. This will create a form of 'withdrawal syndrome' which is caused by decreasing activity in the reward system but also in the mechanisms that provide calm and peace and relaxation. Thereby, the different individuals who are part of a relationship are driven towards each other again to counteract the unease, anxiety and tension.

If the other individual is unavailable, the negative emotions are amplified and the abandoned will try in every way, by searching or perhaps even by force, to get the missing person back. Or they might simply give up and mourn the lost one.

Oxytocin – a key

All of these key aspects of relationships are governed by chemical processes and, as we have described earlier in the book, oxytocin is part of our mammalian heritage and plays a key role in the creation and the maintenance of relationships. Oxytocin has an important function when it comes to getting people to approach each other by increasing the desire to interact and by reducing the fear of others. Oxytocin also facilitates the learning of the other person's characteristics (smell, sound or appearance). Oxytocin is thus not only a mothering hormone but has a much wider function.

Then when the individuals are close to each other a sense of well-being and relaxation is created by oxytocin which activates the reward systems and reduces the activity in the stress systems. After a period of time, the direct closeness is no longer required as the sight or sound or perhaps in the end 'the inner picture' of the other person is enough in order to feel good and to feel calm since the oxytocin-related effects are triggered via the more 'indirect' stimulation.

Our experiences of relationships that we have previously had and those we experience in the present, both positive and negative, have to a certain extent an effect on our future relationships. The more positive relationships we have had, the greater our chances that those in the future will be too.

We are particularly influenced by our early relationships. The more separations we experienced when we were young the more afraid we become about relationships in adulthood and the more painful the separations become. If the relationships early on in life are characterised by calm and trust the greater the chances that relationships in adulthood will be too. This is because the chemical processes involved in the positive or negative experiences of relationships are strengthened. Good relationships early on in life increase, for example, the strength of the oxytocin system.

Drugs and the lack of relationships

But what do people do who do not have any good experiences of relationships and thus find it difficult to socialise with other people? Often life solves the problem by new positive experiences rubbing out the old memories. For some, relationships become a little bit more problematic throughout their lives.

An unfortunate and destructive solution to relationship problems is to use different types of drugs. It is well known that relationship problems may contribute towards some forms of drug abuse. As we have described above, oxytocin plays a key role in relationships, and helps to make us content and happy by activating our reward system and lowering our stress levels. What is actually more natural for those who don't dare or are unable to enter a relationship than to try and get these effects in another way? It may involve alcohol, but also other types of drugs such as cannabis, cocaine or morphine or drugs of the amphetamine type. These drugs have one feature in common with relationships – they activate the body's own reward system, but in a stronger and unnatural or less physiological manner. Therefore, it is easy to become addicted to drugs.

There are, as have been said, many types of drugs which have different effects, some are stimulating whereas others have sedative properties. Ecstasy is a drug which is known to create experiences that are very pleasant and in this world without boundaries everybody seems to be a close friend. New findings show that the 'love hormone' oxytocin, by activating the body's reward system, is a link in the effect chain of ecstasy. The problem is that ecstasy is dangerous, it's addictive and can cause permanent damage to the reward system.

Oxytocin as a medicine

Shouldn't oxytocin be the ideal medicine for individuals who have problems with their relationships? A substance that makes you fearless, social and trusting, that also makes you feel good, and helps you to become calm and relaxed and healthy? There are many people who have problems with their social relationships, perhaps for hereditary reasons or as a consequence of early infections or traumas that have caused autistic tendencies or an extreme fear of other people (social phobia).

The fact is that the dream medicine is actually on its way to becoming a reality and oxytocin is already available as a pharmaceutical. In certain countries such as Sweden, women who are breastfeeding have for a long time been able to receive oxytocin spray if they have had problems with the milk ejection reflex. It has been known that one sniff of synthetic oxytocin gives a high enough level of oxytocin in the blood for the milk to come in. Oxytocin is also used as a medicine when inducing labour or to help stimulate the contractions in slow labour, but it is then administered as a drip.

The oxytocin that is administered as a spray during breastfeeding or as a drip during labour is, from a chemical point of view, completely identical to the oxytocin which is formed in the hypothalamus of mammals, including humans.

Shyness and autism

It is very likely that the oxytocin molecule will be used to lower anxiety, especially in those who are shy or for other reasons have a fear of other people. In many parts of the world, there are ongoing studies showing that oxytocin may actually have a beneficial effect in this context.

Oxytocin's ability to increase social competence is also being tested in individuals with autistic disorders. These individuals find it difficult to understand what other people are feeling. They are also not very good at expressing what they are feeling themselves and are afraid of others. In the clinical trials that are currently under way, researchers deliver oxytocin in the form of a nasal spray and when oxytocin is administered in this way it has a favourable effect on people with autism. They become better at reading other people's emotional states and they become less fearful of them. Studies in which the effect of oxytocin to decrease anxiety and stress levels and alcohol abuse are also being performed.

How should oxytocin be administered?

However, it should be clear that it is not easy to use oxytocin in the form of tablets since the substance is broken down in the gastrointestinal tract. Consequently, a very large quantity is needed and this makes it expensive. Maybe the molecule needs to be modified so that it can survive the environment of the stomach and the intestine and later be absorbed? Another possibility is, of course, that you use nasal spray, as described above. In the worst case scenario oxytocin can be given by injection.

Indirect effects

There are already certain medicines which indirectly utilise the effects of oxytocin. Some of the drugs used to treat schizophrenia, anxiety and depression lead to oxytocin release and oxytocin effects. The oxytocin-releasing drugs include drugs similar to valium and the selective serotonin reuptake inhibitors, the so-called SSRIs, which reduce fear while at the same time increasing social competence. Some of the drugs that are used to treat schizophrenia also increase oxytocin levels and these medicines, in particular, improve the capacity for social interactions. Oxytocin affects the release of other neurotransmitters like serotonin and dopamine and, since these substances also promote oxytocin release, it is difficult to tell which is the chicken and which is the egg, but everything suggests that oxytocin plays a very important role in the effects induced by these drugs.

Problems and dangers

There is, as I see it, a problem with medicines that are based on the oxytocin principle. That is that the substance affects human behaviour in a very profound way and this takes place beyond the control of the conscious mind. With oxytocin, you can create a human who is not only calmer and less scared, but they also become more trusting and generous. These systems are designed to operate in close relationships, where the people involved know each other and, therefore, can trust each other, or in special cases when it is useful to trust an unknown helping person.

The oxytocin-related effects can, on the other hand, cause

some serious problems for a person who is being treated by oxytocin. It is not particularly good to become generous and trusting in the wrong situation. As described earlier in the book, men who had received oxytocin spray invested more money in a computer game than those who hadn't had oxytocin because they trusted their team mates. When they were informed of this and the experiment was carried out again, they still behaved in the same way. The degree of generosity and trust can, so to speak, not be affected by common sense or our conscious will. It is not always good to be too nice. You might regret it afterwards or you might even be taken advantage of by others.

There are several ways to increase the effects of oxytocin. The endogenous oxytocin molecule is very short-lived; it only survives for about twenty minutes in the circulation and maybe slightly longer in the brain. This is probably nature's way of regulating the sensitive mechanisms in the body and in the brain that are affected by oxytocin. In spite of this, experiments are taking place to create oxytocin molecules that can't be broken down as quickly. But it's certainly debateable whether such molecules are only a good thing.

So what happens if the oxytocin molecule is manipulated and becomes much longer lasting? No one knows but the chances are that the effects will become stronger than if you give the natural oxytocin and that it will become even harder for individuals to handle the effects induced as they occur at an unconscious level. One would hope that such substances will not be given to healthy individuals for reasons that are more cosmetic and absolutely not in connection with childbirth and breastfeeding, given the possible long-term effects which could be created – in both the mother and the newborn – on social behaviour and the ability to handle stress. It is, of course, quite a different matter if the substance with enhanced effects is administered to individuals who have an underdeveloped or weak oxytocin system. In this case, this type of substance might be of great value.

The best thing, of course, is to use the body's own oxytocin by activating the release through different types of closeness, touch and perhaps warmth. The endogenous oxytocin cannot be overdosed. Nature has arranged a fine balance between 'reward' and 'withdrawal' when oxytocin is released in short pulses. Also those individuals who normally raise our oxytocin are as a rule, our nearest and dearest and we therefore have reasons to trust them and be generous towards them.

Our oxytocin heritage and society

Our mammalian heritage includes our oxytocin system and the related effects on our social behaviour, our well-being, our calm and our ability to handle stress and also our ability to grow and heal. It is with the aid of oxytocin that we optimise our ability to interact with our parents and our children, but also with other individuals at school and in the workplace. As we have discussed earlier in this book, similar mechanisms operate to hold together both small and large groups. The difference is that the strength of the bond between individuals is more diluted in bigger groups.

We recognise each other, we like being together and we become calm and trusting if a group is functioning as it should. We also need oxytocin as individuals and in our relationships for us to feel good and to be healthy.

But society needs oxytocin too. If we try and discuss oxytocin's effect spectrum from a social perspective, we could say that it contributes towards the unity of the social organism, not through physical closeness but more through common values. When oxytocin prevails, a sense of community and trust is created and therefore a greater understanding of others and thus an openness to negotiation and change. Oxytocin warms and dissolves knots in a 'diplomatic way' without blows or strokes. You could say that oxytocin creates peaceful solutions.

It is helpful to think of the image from one of the stories by the Swedish author Elsa Beskow where you can see Mr

Blue wearing a big homespun coat. Underneath the picture is the question, 'Who can get Mr Blue to take his coat off?' Firstly, a strong wind tries to pull the coat off. The wind does not succeed because Mr Blue just holds the coat closer to his chest. Secondly, the sun comes out and shines on him with its warm rays. And then, Mr Blue gets so warm and feels so good that he removes the coat himself.

Previously, we described how the Rosen Method can be used to create reconciliation between former enemies. When oxytocin is released by closeness and warmth, we can change the inner picture of and the reactions towards the one who touches us.

There are possibly other positive consequences of a high oxytocin level on a societal level. Some researchers, including neuroeconomist Paul Zak from California, say that oxytocin might have positive effects for the economy because it creates trust between humans. If people trust each other, they may invest more in others' companies and sign more agreements and thus you could imagine that economic growth is enhanced. If everyone is scared and holds on to their coat, like Mr Blue, the world will stand still. Paul Zak supports his theory on the basis that in countries where there is greater trust in each other they have a better economy compared to countries where they do not trust each other. But there is virtue in moderation. You mustn't be too generous and gullible either.

In addition, good relationships are beneficial to health in many ways, and not least because positive social relations of any kind increase oxytocin release. As a consequence of this, you get a better ability to balance stress and a reduced risk of developing cardiovascular diseases. The gastrointestinal tract is also protected as we have described earlier and the risk of developing anxiety and depression decreases. Healing and restorative processes are accelerated and learning can be improved. This is obviously also favourable, not only on an individual level, but also on a societal level.

Does our oxytocin heritage get enough stimulation?

The above shows that we should be very keen to protect and cultivate our oxytocin heritage, not only for ourselves and our family's sake, but perhaps also because all of us on earth could live in peace and harmony with each other. Despite this, our oxytocin heritage is exposed to enormous pressures in our time.

It begins at childbirth where the closeness between parents and babies has a positive effect on the oxytocin system's development in both parents and children. Yet this natural contact is prevented in large parts of the world as it is usual to separate the mother and child when the birth happens in a hospital. In Sweden, we have restored the closeness between parents and babies but we instead disturb the early oxytocin-related adaptations with the medical interventions that we provide.

We have described how a mother prepares for motherhood during pregnancy and how the birth with its tremendous increase in oxytocin leads to the mother adapting to motherhood. Because this 'mammalian heritage' is activated, the mother's social competence increases and she becomes more responsive to the child's signals and she knows intuitively how to meet the child. She becomes loving and quickly takes the child to her and feels close. She also becomes calmer but, at the same time, alert to the developments in the environment that could threaten her child.

If the mother and baby then get skin-to-skin contact in the hours after the birth, this first moment of love is enhanced and more or less programmed into both mother and child. As presented before, it was possible after a year to separate the mothers and children who had that early closeness as they had better contact with each other and understood each other better in comparison with mothers and children who had not been close to each other. The mother's sensitivity to the child's signals was greater and the child's ability to stay calm and not become stressed was enhanced. The oxytocin-mediated stimulation of social interaction and calm and peace became permanent because the different hormonal and neurogenic mechanisms that facilitate learning are reinforced during and just after childbirth.

For all modern mothers it is, of course, good that the birth and the early contact with the child make it easier for them to find a good and natural approach towards the child. Perhaps our 'maternal mammalian heritage' is even more important now when new mothers rarely live near their own mothers or other older female relatives? Many mothers of today have not always had access to the information and knowledge about birthing and motherhood, which in the past was orally transmitted from the older women to the younger generation.

Of importance also for the next generation

The strengthening of the capacity for social interaction and the ability to deal with stress which is created in the mother and child by oxytocin in connection with childbirth might not only be of significance for the individual mother but also be important for subsequent generations.

There are reasons to reflect on the rat experiments which showed that the rat pups who received extra care in the form of more touch from their mothers in the first week of life became less scared, more social and more stress-tolerant as adults. This was partly due to the fact that the activity in the pups' oxytocin system had been strengthened. The effects lasted throughout life because certain genes had been activated early in life. But the most important aspect from a generational perspective was that the rats who received extra care when young also became more caring toward their own pups in comparison with the rat mothers who hadn't had the same care. In this way, the good mothering qualities were transferred from one generation to the next. Perhaps newborn babies that receive a lot of closeness early on in life also become more interactive as parents? Perhaps there is also a possibility of generational transfer of our nurturing qualities in our mammalian heritage?

Oxytocin release can be affected

From this standpoint, it might be important to emphasise that the way one gives birth, as well as many of the techniques used for pain relief that are offered to birthing mothers today, may affect oxytocin release during childbirth and therefore possibly also the way mothers interact with their children. It is important to emphasise that women who have had a Caesarean section or an epidural and infusions of oxytocin will still have maternal feelings and will be able to interact with their children. They might have had children before and these skills will already have been stimulated. These feelings will also develop through the oxytocin that is released in the mother's brain in connection with closeness to the child and most of all during breastfeeding.

In an enlightened country like Sweden, where mothers always get to be close to their babies after birth, where they are informed about the importance of closeness and breastfeeding and where they are able to go on maternity leave from their jobs and be at home with their children for a very long time, perhaps the negative impact of a possible lack of oxytocin during childbirth is counteracted.

But what happens in countries where mothers may not be close to their babies after birth, do not breastfeed and in addition have to go back to work almost immediately? Are we going to see different types of mothers under such circumstances? And thus, in the longer run, different kinds of children? This is something to reflect on, particularly as it is becoming much more common in many countries to give birth by Caesarean section or to have an epidural and an oxytocin drip in connection with vaginal birth.

It is perhaps on the societal level that the consequences of the lack of oxytocin stimulation should be studied. You can imagine that there might be a slight weakness of the maternal adaptations and hence the child's capacity for social relationships and love and perhaps even the ability to handle stress and pain. If these abilities don't get 'nudged' at birth, what will then happen to the human race after ten, a hundred or a thousand generations? The risk is that the human oxytocin-related psychological and physiological abilities weaken. What would then happen to humanity and the ability to love and co-operate within the family, in the workplace, within the country and between countries?

Can we in our world afford not to use this natural stimulus of the good forces within us that the birth-related oxytocin release provides?

The disintegrated family

The closeness between parents and children may not always be to the maximum during the first years of life, not least for practical reasons since time might be insufficient when both parents are working. Overall, the role of the family has become less important and separations are more common. We are encouraged by our culture, and women especially, to be independent, hardworking and successful. This sometimes happens at the expense of relationships. Many people live the single life, not least in the big cities, though many of them do not really want to live that way. With the trend for smaller families, many people spend their old age in great loneliness at home or in a retirement home.

Apart from the parents, grandparents, siblings and other relatives have always been an important base and safety factor for most people throughout their lives. In our time and culture, the big families, where the grandparents, siblings and other relatives lived together, have more or less disappeared. People also often live in other configurations other than the classical pair or the nuclear family. Often the biological parents are complemented with 'bonus parents', nursery teachers or other important significant people. It is believed that through repeated contact with the same person or persons, over time the security system in the children is developed whether they are relatives or not. The main thing is that there is consistency in the availability and regularity in the relations.

Reduced closeness in the
family a reason for insecurity?

It may after all be reasonable to ask the questions if the above-described changes in the family structure and living patterns to some extent affect the contemporary human's well-being and security. We have a high standard of living, we eat and live well. Most children have their own bedrooms and perhaps their own TV or computer. All of them get to go to school and most adults work during large parts of their lives.

We can get healthcare when we are sick. Tuberculosis and other infections have become rare due to the reduction in overcrowding and improved standards of hygiene. Despite this, there is an increase in mental illness. Young women in particular find it a struggle. There are many who feel empty, insecure and rootless, despite the high material standards and perhaps successes in their studies and in their careers.

There are, of course, many explanations for this. The stress level has increased exponentially in the last few decades. Phones are ringing everywhere and via e-mail and other communications you can be reached by many people anywhere and at any time of day. Everyone needs to find time for everything: work, family and leisure. But this equation does not work for everyone. Some of us collapse because the demands and the pace are simply too high.

But could there be yet another factor behind this new insecurity? Perhaps there were invisible positive effects of having fewer financial resources, living in a large family and being overcrowded? Perhaps the touch-related security system was activated more strongly in the children who lived in the same room as their parents or siblings, and maybe even sharing a bed with them for many years? To always have someone close when being young was perhaps not just a nuisance? Perhaps the overcrowding and lack of modern technology created an abundance of closeness, warmth and touch which gave rise to a kind of basic security that no material abundance or any professional success later in life can ever create?

The automated and anonymous workplace

It is not only in the family that there have been major changes. The working climate has also intensified in many workplaces. The pace has increased and a lot of the time, work is carried out individually together with a computer. The relationship to the computer, an often much loved thing, or the individuals with whom you communicate via the computer, is after all different compared to the relationship you have with people who are in the same room, because then all the senses are involved in the communication.

The time when long talks took place in the coffee room is over. There is no time for that. Better to take the coffee from the vending machine and drink it at your desk together with the computer. When the competition is intense and job security low, it is natural to push ahead, sometimes possibly even at the expense of others. This also contributes towards an increase in loneliness.

During each reorganisation, chaos is created and if you are unable to understand why and if it is not anchored across the board, this natural feeling of loneliness and alienation is reinforced in many employees. If there is also no appreciation or support from the managers, it is easy to be drained of the positive oxytocin forces. On the other hand, if you are being seen and appreciated for what you do and understand your work to be meaningful, you're willing to work as much as needed. In many workplaces, they are starting to realise that a good oxytocin climate is extremely important for unity, satisfaction and hence job performance and they work actively to support these aspects.

How do we protect our oxytocin heritage?

If by now we realise that it is important to nurture our oxytocin system so that it is not damaged by the reduction of time for relationships, by all the stress and all the demands that drive us towards self-sufficiency, competition and independence, what do we need to do?

The most important thing is to increase our knowledge about the oxytocin system that makes us feel better and have better relationships in both our small worlds and in the big world. We should thus be aware that our modern lifestyle can damage our invisible oxytocin heritage, because much of the closeness which was automatically provided in the past has disappeared. But we can also learn about the ways in which each and every one of us can help to increase its effects.

It obviously starts with childbirth. The closeness between parents and child is incredibly important and if the immediate contact is prevented because of a Caesarean section or some form of anaesthesia, you can compensate for this by offering extra closeness in the time after.

Touch in any form is good and enhances the development of the oxytocin system. This is known by most, but perhaps it is just a matter of sitting next to your children while they're watching the TV and perhaps also massaging their backs for a while before they go to sleep. It is easy to lose the closeness when the children get older. It is, in fact, not much that is needed.

In the study that we referred to earlier in the book, in which children at nursery received extra massage during rest times, clear effects were visible after six months of treatment, even though the children might only have received massage for ten minutes. Obviously, relatively short periods of extra touch are sufficient, as long as they occur fairly frequently and regularly.

Another conclusion to be drawn from these results is that our daily natural supply of closeness must be quite small. Otherwise, a short period of extra touch for as few as ten minutes a day would not be sufficient to be able to produce such positive effects on the children's behaviour. Without us noticing and without us having bad intentions, the closeness account has been emptied by the changes in our lifestyle. Our skin hunger is simply not full up!

In preschools and nurseries, various types of massage

which the children give to each other have been introduced in many places. This has often resulted in excellent results and will surely be used more, perhaps even in school. Of course, it needs to be done using very gentle types of massage with great care and strict rules.

As an adult, allowing yourself to be touched or massaged at times by someone who really knows how to do it, is not a bad idea. In elderly care, in the hospice and even within emergency and intensive care units, patients have started to be provided with touch or soft massage. Many of the touch-hungry elderly and the sick not only enjoy the nice moment but also become more alert and less anxious. The relationship between the staff and the patient is also improved because both of them are affected. We will most certainly see much more of touch therapies within the care industry in the future.

To get your hair or skin done at the hairdresser's or skin therapist and massage yourself with scented creams is not only nice but also healthy. It might not always be additional people involved. To a certain extent, you can help your own oxytocin by nurturing and taking care of your own skin and body.

Perhaps we should have a dog or another pet at home that meets the children if they come home from school before mum and dad have returned from work? There are many studies showing that children do improve their social competence if they have a pet and also their ability to concentrate, for example, when doing their homework, as we saw earlier. It is easier to do homework when someone is at home and it's not so empty. To ride and take care of horses also develops the ability to relate and is very sought after, especially by teenage girls.

To swim and bathe and to be in the (not too strong) sun is also nice and touching and gives many people great pleasure. It is also healing to be out in nature and many people feel much better by spending time working in a garden setting. This stimulates many of the senses through the touching of plants and the soil, but of course also by the sensory stimulation from the sun and wind and the thoughts and fantasies about the plants' beauty and eternal life cycle. Severe fatigue reactions can be helped with horticultural therapy, as has been demonstrated by Patrik Grahn and Inga-Lena Bengtsson at the Swedish University of Agricultural Sciences.

It is beneficial to be physically active or to just walk and hold a conversation. Dancing, and in particular dancing with a partner, is described by many as an excellent way to feel good and joyful, both through the movement and through the closeness.

It is important to remember to do things together and not always sitting alone at the computer. To listen to music, go to the theatre, go to church, read books or look at art bring so much goodness and can certainly to some extent aid oxytocin. To sing in a choir has been shown to increase levels of oxytocin and is described by many as a source of great joy and a sense of community.

Perhaps diet also plays a role for oxytocin? Warm food is probably better than cold and foods that contain fat and protein increase oxytocin release more than carbohydrates. Another reason not to remove fat from the diet. According to neuroeconomist Paul Zak, people who eat a lot of soya beans, which contain plant oestrogens which affect oxytocin, are better at resolving conflicts.

Thus, there are plenty of small steps one can take. It depends to some extent on who you are and also on how you live. The key is to be aware that touch and closeness are important. Perhaps in the future, small devices will be developed, similar to those that count your steps, so that you can register and see if you meet your touch and closeness needs? Perhaps doctors in the future will prescribe touch in the same way as they prescribe exercise?

The message of this book is that oxytocin is important for us to feel good, to be healthy and to make our relationships work well. Our oxytocin is nourished by closeness. By nurturing and cultivating our oxytocin heritage, we can improve not only our own relationships in the local community but also those from a societal perspective. When the feeling of community is strengthened, we increase the chances of finding peaceful solutions for conflicts and we can work together to assume a joint responsibility for the care of our earth's resources.

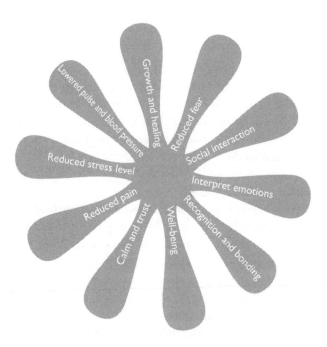

The oxytocin flower. The various petals represent the different effects that oxytocin may bring, in the context of closeness and relationships.

Acknowledgements

When writing a book like this, you do not do it on your own. There are many who have contributed to the internal knowledge base and the synthesis of knowledge on which this book is based. In the first instance, it's about my colleagues on all different levels, that is, from my own supervisors and mentors and to those I supervised and tried to educate and develop, but of course also about all my other colleagues and co-workers. I thank you all!

There is another group of scientists and people that I would like to acknowledge who have been important to enable this book to be written, and these are those who think broadly and see the connections and not just the details. The latter have increased in medical research in recent years because so much research is based on studies of genes, molecules and on the individual cell's functions, which has contributed to the explosion of medical and biological research. I have my roots in another, today almost extinct tradition of research where we are more interested in the whole organism and its entirety.

Paradoxically, it is this knowledge or ability that you need today because the focus is slowly shifting towards wholeness and context again. This is particularly important because it is with this perspective in mind that we can build bridges between the different scientific disciplines, and thus understand that all knowledge that comes from different traditions do in fact derive from the same elephant, even if you might be using the tail or the ears to see with. I am deeply grateful to those who have taught me to think holistically and in context.

References

1. Our mammalian heritage

Algers, B. et al. (1991). Quantitative relationships between suckling-induced teat stimulation and the release of prolactin, gastrin, somatostatin, insulin, glucagon and vasoactive intestinal polypeptide in sows. *Veterinary Research Communications*, 15, 395–407.

Algers, B. & Uvnäs Moberg, K. (2007). Maternal behavior in pigs. *Hormones and Behavior*, 52, 78–85.

Bielsky, I. F. & Young, L. J. (2004). Oxytocin, vasopressin, and social recognition in mammals. *Peptides*, 25, 1565–74.

Bosch, O. J. et al. (2005). Brain oxytocin correlates with maternal aggression: link to anxiety. *The Journal of Neuroscience*, 20, 6807–15.

Broad, K. D., Curley, J. P. & Keverne, E. B. (2006). Mother–infant bonding and the evolution of mammalian social relationships. *Philosophical Transactions of the Royal Society B: Biological Sciences*, 29, 2199–214.

Cameron, N. M. et al. (2008). Epigenetic programming of phenotypic variations in reproductive strategies in the rat through maternal care. *Journal of Neuroendocrinology*, 20, 975–801.

DeVries, A. C., Taymans, S. E. & Carter, C. S. (1997). Social modulation of corticosteroid responses in male prairie voles. *Annals of the New York Academy of Sciences*, 807, 494–7.

Hofer, M. A. (1994). Early relationships as regulators of infant physiology and behaviour. *Acta Paediatrica Supplement*, 397, 9–18.

Holst, S., Uvnäs Moberg, K. & Petersson, M. (2002). Postnatal oxytocin treatment and postnatal stroking of rats reduce blood pressure in adulthood. *Autonomic Neuroscience*, 30, 85–90.

Kendrick, K. M. et al. (1997). Neural control of maternal behaviour and olfactory recognition of offspring. *Brain Research Bulletin*, 44, 383–95.

Kendrick, K. M., Lévy, F. & Keverne, E. B. (1991). Importance of vaginocervical stimulation for the formation of maternal bonding in primiparous and multiparous parturient ewes. *Physiology & Behavior*, 50, 595–600.

Keverne, E. B. & Curley, J. P. (2004). Vasopressin, oxytocin and social behaviour. *Current Opinion in Neurobiology*, 14, 777–83.

Keverne, E. B. & Kendrick, K. M. (1994). Maternal behaviour in sheep and its neuroendocrine regulation. *Acta Paediatrica Supplement*, 397, 47–56.

Landgraf, R. et al. (2003). Viral vector-mediated gene transfer of the vole V1a vasopressin receptor in the rat septum: improved social discrimination and active social behaviour. *European Journal of Neuroscience*, 18, 403–11.

Lonstein, J. S. (2005). Reduced anxiety in postpartum rats requires recent physical interactions with pups, but is independent of suckling and peripheral sources of hormones. *Hormones and Behavior*, 47, 241–55.

Martel, F. L. et al. (1993). Opioid receptor blockade reduces maternal affect and social grooming in rhesus monkeys. *Psychoneuroendocrinology*, 18, 307–21.

Martel, F. L. et al. (1995). Effects of opioid receptor blockade on the social behavior of rhesus monkeys living in large family groups. *Developmental Psychobiology*, 28, 71–84.

Neumann, I. D. (2008). Brain oxytocin: a key regulator of emotional and social behaviours in both females and males. *Journal of Neuroendocrinology*, 20, 858–65.

Nowak, R. et al. (1997). Cholecystokinin receptors mediate the development of a preference for the mother by newly born lambs. *Behavior & Neuroscience*, 111, 1375–82.

Nowak, R. et al. (1997). Development of a preferential relationship with the mother by the newborn lamb: importance of the sucking activity. *Physiology & Behavior*, 62, 681–8.

Uvnäs Moberg, K. (1998). Oxytocin may mediate the benefits of positive social interaction and emotions. *Psychoneuroendocrinology*, 23, 819–35. Review.

Waldherr, M. & Neumann, I. D. (2007). Centrally released oxytocin mediates mating-induced anxiolysis in male rats. *Proceedings of the National Academy of Sciences of the United States of America*, 104, 16681–4.

Weller, L. & Weller, A. (2002). Menstrual synchrony and cycle variability: a reply to Schank (2000). *Psychoneuroendocrinology*, 27, 519–26.

Williams, J. R. et al. (1994). Oxytocin administered centrally facilitates formation of a partner preference in female prairie voles (Microtus ochrogaster). *Journal of Neuroendocrinology*, 6, 247–50.

Winslow, J. T. et al. (1993). A role for central vasopressin in pair bonding in monogamous prairie voles. *Nature*, 365, 545–8.

Ågren, G. et al. (1997). Olfactory cues from an oxytocin-injected male rat can reduce energy loss in its cagemates. *Neuroreport*, 28, 2551–5.

Ågren, G., Uvnäs Moberg, K. & Lundeberg, T. (1997). Olfactory cues from an oxytocin-injected male rat can induce anti-nociception in its cagemates. *Neuroreport*, 29, 3073–6.

2. Closeness and attachment

Ainsworth, M. D. (1985). Patterns of infant–mother attachments: antecedents and effects on development. *Bulletin of the New York Academy of Medicine*, 61, 771–791.

Bowlby, J. (1969). *Attachment and loss: Volume 1: Attachment*. New York: Basic Books.

Bowlby, J. (1973). *Attachment and loss: Volume 2: Separation*. New York: Basic Books.

Bowlby, J. (1980). *Attachment and loss: Volume 3: Loss: Sadness and Depression*. New York: Basic Books.

Broberg, A. et al. (2006). *Anknytningsteori. Betydelsen av nära känslomässiga relationer*. Stockholm: Natur & Kultur.

Broberg, A. et al. (2008). *Anknytning i praktiken. Tillämpningar av anknytningsteorin.* Stockholm: Natur & Kultur.

Bystrova, K. et al. (2009). Early contact versus separation: Effects on mother–infant interaction one year later. *Birth.*

Champagne, F. A. & Meaney, M. J. (2008). Transgenerational effects of social environment on variations in maternal care and behavioral response to novelty. *Behavior & Neuroscience,* 121, 1353–1363.

Francis, D. D., Champagne, F. C. & Meaney, M. J. (2000). Variations in maternal behaviour are associated with differences in oxytocin receptor levels in the rat. *Journal of Neuroendocrinology,* 12, 1145–1148.

Harlow, H. F., Rowland, G. L. & Griffin, G. A. (1964). The effect of total social deprivation on the development of monkey behavior. *Psychiatric Research Report of the American Psychiatric Association,* 19, 116–135.

Klaus, M. H. et al. (1972). Maternal attachment. Importance of the first post-partum days. *The New England Journal of Medicine,* 286, 460–463.

Lorenz, K. (1935/1957). Companionship in birdlife. In C. H. Schiller (ed.), *Instinctive Behaviour.* New York: International Universities Press.

Lorenz, K. (1963). *King Solomon's ring: New light on animal ways.* London: Routledge.

Pavlov, I. P. (1951). *Conditioned reflex.* 10, 3–10.

Pavlov, I. P. (1951). *Conditioned reflex.* 11, 6–12.

Seay, B., Alexander, B. K. & Harlow, H. F. (1964). Maternal behavior of socially deprived rhesus monkeys. *Journal of Abnormal Psychology,* 69, 345–354.

Spinelli, S. et al. (2007). Association between the recombinant human serotonin transporter linked promoter region polymorphism and behavior in rhesus macaques during a separation paradigm. *Development in Psychopathology,* 19, 977–987.

Suomi, S. J., van der Horst, F. C. & van der Veer, R. (2008). Rigorous experiments on monkey love: an account of Harry F. Harlow's role in the history of Attachment Theory. *Integrative Psychological and Behavioral Science,* 42, 354–369.

3. How is the body controlled?

Araki, T. et al. (1984). Responses of adrenal sympathetic nerve activity and catecholamine secretion to cutaneous stimulation in anesthetized rats. *Neuroscience,* 12, 231–237.

Björkstrand, E. et al. (1990). Suckling-induced release of cholecystokinin into plasma in the lactating rat: effects of abdominal vagotomy and lesions of central pathways concerned with milk ejection. *Journal of Endocrinology,* 127, 257–263.

Craig, A. D. (2003). Pain mechanisms: labeled lines versus convergence in central processing. *Annual Review of Neuroscience,* 26, 1–30.

Eriksson, M. et al. (1994). Role of vagal nerve activity during suckling. Effects on plasma levels of oxytocin, prolactin, VIP, somatostatin, insulin, glucagon, glucose and of milk secretion in lactating rats. *Acta Physiologica Scandinavica,* 151, 453–459.

Eriksson, M. et al. (1996). Distribution and origin of peptide-containing nerve fibres in the rat and human mammary gland. *Neuroscience,* 70, 227–45.

Eriksson, M., Lundeberg, T. & Uvnäs Moberg, K. (1996). Studies on cutaneous blood flow in the mammary gland of lactating rats. *Acta Physiologica Scandinavica*, 158, 1–6.

Guyton, A. (1991). *Textbook of medical physiology* (8th edition, chapter X). Philadelphia: WB Saunders.

Holst, S. et al. (2005). Massage-like stroking influences plasma levels of gastrointestinal hormones, including insulin, and increases weight gain in male rats. *Autonomic Neuroscience*, 120, 73–9.

Kurosawa, M. et al. (1995). Massage-like stroking of the abdomen lowers blood pressure in anesthetized rats: influence of oxytocin. *Journal of the Autonomic Nervous System*, 56, 26–30.

Lund, I. et al. (1999). Sensory stimulation (massage) reduces blood pressure in unanaesthetized rats. *Journal of the Autonomic Nervous System*, 78, 30–37.

Lund, I et al. (2002). Repeated massage-like stimulation induces long-term effects on nociception: contribution of oxytocinergic mechanisms. *European Journal of Neuroscience*, 16, 330–338.

Montagu, A. (1986). *Touching: the human significance of the skin* (3rd edition). New York: Harper and Row.

Olausson, H. W. et al. (2008). Unmyelinated tactile afferents have opposite effects on insular and somatosensory cortical processing. *Neuroscience Letters*, 436, 128–132.

Olausson, H. W. et al. The neurophysiology of unmyelinated tactile afferents. *Neuroscience & Biobehavioral Review*.

Sato, A. (1987). Neural mechanisms of somatic sensory regulation of catecholamine secretion from the adrenal gland. *Advances in Biophysical Research*, 23, 905–926.

Sivamani, R. K. et al. (2009). The benefits and risks of ultraviolet tanning and its alternatives: the role of prudent sun exposure. *Dermatologic Clinics*, 27, 149–54.

Stock, S. & Uvnäs Moberg, K. (1988). Increased plasma levels of oxytocin in response to afferent electrical stimulation of the sciatic and vagal nerves and in response to touch and pinch in anaesthetized rats. *Acta Physiologica Scandinavica*, 132, 29–34.

Uvnäs Moberg, K. (2011). *The Oxytocin Factor: Tapping the hormone of calm, love and healing.* London: Pinter & Martin.

Uvnäs Moberg, K. et al. (1985). Plasma levels of oxytocin increase in response to suckling and feeding in dogs and sows. *Acta Physiologica Scandinavica*, 124, 391–398.

Uvnäs Moberg, K. et al. (1992). Vagally mediated release of gastrin and cholecystokinin following sensory stimulation. *Acta Physiologica Scandinavica*, 146, 349–56.

Uvnäs Moberg, K. et al. (1993). The antinociceptive effect of non-noxious sensory stimulation is mediated partly through oxytocinergic mechanisms. *Acta Physiologica Scandinavica*, 149, 199–204.

Uvnäs Moberg, K. et al. (1996). Stroking of the abdomen causes decreased locomotor activity in conscious male rats. *Physiology & Behavior*, 60, 1409–11.

Uvnäs-Moberg, K. & Eriksson, M. (1983). Release of gastrin and insulin in response to suckling in lactating dogs. *Acta Physiologica Scandinavica*, 119, 181–185.

Uvnäs-Moberg, K. & Eriksson, M. (1996). Breastfeeding: physiological, endocrine and behavioural adaptations caused by oxytocin and local neurogenic activity in the nipple and mammary gland (Review). *Acta Paediatrica*, 85, 525–530.

Währborg, P. (1989). *Stress och den nya ohälsan*. Stockholm: Natur & Kultur.

Ågren, G. et al. (1995). The oxytocin antagonist 1 – deamino -2D Tyr-(Oet)- 4-Thr-8-Orn-oxytocin reverses the increase in withdrawal response latency to thermal, but not mechanical, nociceptive stimuli following oxytocin administration or massage-like stroking in rats. *Neuroscience Letters*, 187, 49–52.

4. What is oxytocin?

Acher, A., Chauvet, J. & Chauvet, M. T. (1995). Man and the chimaera: selective versus neutral oxytocin evolution. In R. Ivell & J. A. Russell (eds.) *Oxytocin: cellular and molecular approaches in medicine and research* (s. 615–617). New York: Plenum Press.

Argiolas, A. & Gessa, G. L. (1991). Central functions of oxytocin. *Neuroscience & Biobehavioural Reviews*, 15, 217–231.

Baumgartner, T. et al. (2008). Oxytocin shapes the neural circuitry of trust and trust adaptation in humans. *Neuron*, 58, 639–50.

Bielsky, I. F. & Young, L. J. (2004). Oxytocin, vasopressin, and social recognition in mammals. *Peptides*, 25, 1565–74.

Dale, H. H. (1906). On some physiological actions of ergot. *The Journal of Physiology*, 34, 163–206.

Díaz-Cabiale, Z. et al. (2000). Systemic oxytocin treatment modulates alpha 2-adrenoceptors in telencephalic and diencephalic regions of the rat. *Brain Research*, 887, 421–425.

Ditzen, B. et al. (2009). Intranasal oxytocin increases positive communication and reduces cortisol levels during couple conflict. *Biological Psychiatry*, 95, 728–31.

Domes, G. et al. (2007). Oxytocin improves "mind-reading" in humans. *Biological Psychiatry*, 61, 731–733.

Domes, G. et al. (2007). Oxytocin attenuates amygdala responses to emotional faces regardless of valence. *Biological Psychiatry*, 62, 1187–1190.

Gimpl, G. & Fahrenholz, F. (2001). The oxytocin receptor system: structure, function, and regulation (review). *Physiological Review*, 81, 629–683.

Guyton, A. (1991). *Textbook of medical physiology* (8th edition, chapter X). Philadelphia: WB Saunders.

Holst, S., Uvnäs Moberg, K. & Petersson, M. (2002). Postnatal oxytocin treatment and postnatal stroking of rats reduce blood pressure in adulthood. *Autonomic Neuroscience*, 99, 85–90.

Kirsch, P. et al. (2005). Oxytocin modulates neural circuitry for social cognition and fear in humans. *Journal of Neuroscience*, 25, 11489–11493.

Kosfeld, M. et al. (2005). Oxytocin increases trust in humans. *Nature*, 435, 673–676.

Ludwig, M. et al. (2002). The active role of dendrites in the regulation of magnocellular neurosecretory cell behavior (review). *Progress in Brain Research*, 139, 247–256.

Neumann, I. D. et al. (2000). Brain oxytocin inhibits basal and stress-induced activity of the hypothalamo-pituitary-adrenal axis in male and female rats: partial action within the paraventricular nucleus. *Journal of Neuroendocrinology*, 12, 235–243.

Ott, I. & Scott, J. C. (1910). The action of infundibulum upon the mammary secretion. *Proceedings of the Society for Experimental Biology and Medicine*, 8, 137–142.

Petersson, M. et al. (1996). Oxytocin causes a long-term decrease of blood pressure in female and male rats. *Physiology & Behavior*, 60, 1311–5.

Petersson, M. et al. (1996). Oxytocin increases nociceptive thresholds in a longterm perspective in female and male rats. *Neuroscience Letters*, 212, 87–90.

Petersson, M. et al. (1998). Oxytocin increases locus coeruleus alpha 2-adrenoreceptor responsiveness in rats. *Neuroscience Letters*, 255, 115–8.

Petersson, M. et al. (1998). Oxytocin increases the survival of musculocutaneous flaps. *Naunyn-Schmiedeberg's Archives of Pharmacology*, 357, 701–4.

Petersson, M. et al. (1999). Long-term changes in gastrin, cholecystokinin and insulin in response to oxytocin treatment. *Neuroendocrinology*, 69, 202–8.

Petersson, M. & Uvnäs Moberg, K. (2003). Systemic oxytocin treatment modulates glucocorticoid and mineralocorticoid receptor mRNA in the rat hippocampus. *Neuroscience Letters*, 343, 97–100.

Petersson, M. & Uvnäs Moberg, K. (2004). Prolyl-leucyl-glycinamide shares some effects with oxytocin but decreases oxytocin levels. *Physiology & Behavior*, 83, 475–81.

Petersson, M. & Uvnäs Moberg, K. (2007). Effects of an acute stressor on blood pressure and heart rate in rats pretreated with intracerebroventricular oxytocin injections. *Psychoneuroendocrinology*, 32, 959–965.

Petersson, M., Hulting, A. L. & Uvnäs Moberg, K. (1999). Oxytocin causes a sustained decrease in plasma levels of corticosterone in rats. *Neuroscience Letters*, 264, 41–44.

Petersson, M., Lundeberg, T. & Uvnäs Moberg, K. (1999). Oxytocin enhances the effects of clonidine on blood pressure and locomotor activity in rats. *Journal of the Autonomic Nervous System*, 78, 49–56.

Richard, P., Moos, F. & Freund-Mercier, M. J. (1991). Central effects of oxytocin. *Physiological Review*, 71, 331–370.

Russell, J. A., Leng, G. & Douglas, A. J. (2003). The magnocellular oxytocin system, the fount of maternity: adaptations in pregnancy. *Frontiers in Neuroendocrinology*, 24, 27–61.

Skuse, D. H. & Gallagher, L. (2009). Dopaminergic-neuropeptide interactions in the social brain. *Trends in Cognitive Sciences*, 13, 27–35.

Sofroniew, M. W. (1983). Vasopressin and oxytocin in mammalian brain and spinal cord. *Trends in Neurosciences*, 6, 467–472.

Uvnäs Moberg, K. (1997). Oxytocin linked antistress effects – the relaxation and growth response (review). *Acta Physiologica Scandinavica Supplement*, 640, 38–42.

Uvnäs Moberg, K. (1998). Antistress Pattern Induced by Oxytocin. *News in Physiological Sciences*, 13, 22–25.

Uvnäs Moberg, K. et al. (1994). High doses of oxytocin cause sedation and low doses cause an anxiolytic-like effect in male rats. *Pharmacology, Biochemistry & Behaviour*, 49, 101–106.

Uvnäs Moberg, K. et al. (1995). Suggestive evidence for a DA D3 receptor-mediated increase in the release of oxytocin in the male rat. *Neuroreport*, 6, 1338–40.

Uvnäs Moberg, K. et al. (1996). Effects of 5-HT agonists, selective for different receptor subtypes, on oxytocin, CCK, gastrin and somatostatin plasma levels in the rat. *Neuropharmacology*, 35, 1635–40.

Uvnäs Moberg, K. et al. (1998). Postnatal oxytocin injections cause sustained weight gain and increased nociceptive thresholds in male and female rats. *Pediatric Research*, 43, 344–348.

Uvnäs Moberg, K. et al. (2000). Improved conditioned avoidance learning by oxytocin administration in high emotional but not low emotional Sprague Dawley rats. *Regulatory Peptides*, 88, 27–32.

Uvnäs Moberg, K. & Petersson, M. (2004). Oxytocin–biochemical link for human relations. Mediator of antistress, well-being, social interaction, growth, healing. *Läkartidningen*, 101, 2634–2639.

Uvnäs Moberg, K. & Petersson, M. (2005). Oxytocin, a mediator of antistress, well-being, social interaction, growth and Healing. *Zeitschrift fur Psychosomatische Medizin und Psychotherapie*, 51, 57–80.

Wakerley, J. B. & Ingram, C. D. (1993). Synchronization of bursting in hypothalamic oxytocin neurons: Possible coordinating mechanisms. *News in Physiological Sciences*, 8, 129–133.

Williams, J. R. et al. (1994). Oxytocin administered centrally facilitates formation of a partner preference in female prairie voles (Microtus ochrogaster). *Journal of Neuroendocrinology*, 6, 247–50.

Winslow, J. T. et al. (1993). A role for central vasopressin in pair bonding in monogamous prairie voles. *Nature*, 365, 545–8.

5. Oxytocin and attachment

Bosch, O. J. et al. (2005). Brain oxytocin correlates with maternal aggression: link to anxiety. *Journal of Neuroscience*, 25, 6807–6815.

Broad, K. D. et al. (1999). Previous maternal experience potentiates the effect of parturition on oxytocin receptor mRNA expression in the paraventricular nucleus. *European Journal of Neuroscience*, 11, 3725–37.

Bystrova, K. et al. (2003). Skin-to-skin contact may reduce negative consequences of "the stress of being born": a study on temperature in newborn infants, subjected to different ward routines in St. Petersburg. *Acta Paediatrica*, 92, 320–326.

Bystrova, K. et al. (2007). Maternal axillar and breast temperature after giving birth: effects of delivery ward practices and relation to infant temperature. *Birth*, 34, 291–300.

Bystrova, K. et al. (2007). The effect of Russian Maternity Home routines on breastfeeding and neonatal weight loss with special reference to swaddling. *Early Human Development*, 83, 29–39.

Bystrova, K. et al. (2009). Early contact versus separation: Effects on mother–infant interaction one year later. *Birth*, 36, 97–109.

Cameron, N. M. et al. (2008). Epigenetic programming of phenotypic variations in reproductive strategies in the rat through maternal care. *Journal of Neuroendocrinology*, 20, 975–801.

Champagne, F. A. & Meaney, M. J. (2007). Transgenerational effects of social environment on variations in maternal care and behavioral response to novelty. *Behavioral Neuroscience*, 121, 1353–1363.

Christensson, K. et al. (1995). Separation distress call in the human neonate in the absence of maternal body contact. *Acta Paediatrica*, 84, 468–73.

Erlandsson, K. et al. (2007). Skin-to-skin care with the father after cesarean birth and its effect on newborn crying and prefeeding behavior. *Birth*, 34, 105–14.

Febo, M., Numan, M. & Ferris, C. F. (2005). Functional magnetic resonance imaging shows oxytocin activates brain regions associated with mother-pup bonding during suckling. *Journal of Neuroscience*, 25, 11637–11644.

Feldman, R. (2004). Mother–infant skin-to-skin contact (Kangaroo Care). Theoretical, clinical and empirical aspects. *Infants and Young Children*, 17, 145–161.

Feldman, R. et al. (2007). Evidence for a neuroendocrinological foundation of human affiliation: plasma oxytocin levels across pregnancy and the postpartum period predict mother–infant bonding. *Psychological Science*, 18, 965–970.

Francis, D. D., Champagne, F. C. & Meaney, M. J. (2000). Variations in maternal behaviour are associated with differences in oxytocin receptor levels in the rat. *Journal of Neuroendocrinology*, 12, 1145–1148.

Gillath, O. et al. (2008). Genetic correlates of adult attachment style. *Personality and Social Psychology Bulletin*, 34, 1396–1405.

Gordon, I. et al. (2008). Oxytocin and cortisol in romantically unattached young adults: associations with bonding and psychological distress. *Psychophysiology*, 45, 349–352.

Gray, P. B., Yang, C. F. & Pope, H. G. Jr. (2006). Fathers have lower salivary testosterone levels than unmarried men and married non-fathers in Beijing, China. Proceedings. *Biological Sciences*, 273, 333–339.

Harlow, H. F., Rowland, G. L. & Griffin, G. A. (1964). The effect of total social deprivation on the development of monkey behavior. *Psychiatric Research Report of the American Psychiatric Association*, 19, 116–135.

Hofer, M. A. (1994). Early relationships as regulators of infant physiology and behaviour. *Acta Paediatrica Supplement*, 397, 9–18.

Jonas, W. et al. (2007). Newborn skin temperature two days postpartum during breastfeeding related to different labour ward practices. *Early Human Development* 2007: 83, 55–62.

Jonas, W. et al. (2008). Influence of oxytocin or epidural analgesia on personality profile in breastfeeding women: a comparative study. *Archives of Women's Mental Health*, 11, 335–45.

Jonas, W. et al. (2008). Short- and long-term decrease of blood pressure in women during breastfeeding. *Breastfeeding Medicine*, 3, 103–9.

Jonas, W. et al. Effects of medical interventions during labor and the perinatal period on the release of oxytocin and prolactin in response to breastfeeding two days after birth. *Breastfeeding Medicine*.

Kendrick, K. M. et al. (1997). Neural control of maternal behaviour and olfactory recognition of offspring. *Brain Research Bulletin*, 44, 383–95.

Kendrick, K. M., Lévy, F. & Keverne, E. B. (1991). Importance of vaginocervical stimulation for the formation of maternal bonding in primiparous and multiparous parturient ewes. *Physiology & Behavior*, 50, 595–600.

Keverne, E. B. & Curley, J. P. (2004). Vasopressin, oxytocin and social behaviour. *Current Opinion in Neurobiology*, 14, 777–83.

Keverne, E. B. & Kendrick, K. M. (1994). Maternal behaviour in sheep and its neuroendocrine regulation. *Acta Paediatrica Supplement*, 397, 47–56.

Klaus, M. H. et al. (1972). Maternal attachment. Importance of the first post-partum days. *New England Journal of Medicine*, 286, 460–463.

Klaus, M. H. & Klaus, P. H. (1998). *Your amazing newborn*. Massachusetts: Perseus Books.

Lee, S. Y. et al. (2005). Does long-term lactation protect premenopausal women against hypertension risk? A Korean women's cohort study. *Preventive Medicine*, 41, 433–438.

Levine, A. et al. Oxytocin during pregnancy and early postpartum: individual patterns and maternal-fetal attachment. *Peptides*, 28, 1162–1169.

Lonstein, J. S. (2005). Reduced anxiety in postpartum rats requires recent physical interactions with pups, but is independent of suckling and peripheral sources of hormones. *Hormones & Behavior*, 47, 241–55.

Marazziti, D. et al. (2006). A relationship between oxytocin and anxiety of romantic attachment. *Clinical Practice and Epidemiology in Mental Health*, 11, 28.

Matthiesen, A. S. et al. (2001). Postpartum maternal oxytocin release by newborns: effects of infant hand massage and sucking. *Birth*, 28, 13–9.

Meinlschmidt, G. & Heim, C. (2007). Sensitivity to intranasal oxytocin in adult men with early parental separation. *Biological Psychiatry*, 61, 1109–1111.

Nelson, E. E. & Panksepp, J. (1998). Brain substrates of infant–mother attachment: contributions of opioids, oxytocin, and norepinephrine (review). *Neuroscience & Biobehavioral Reviews*, 22, 437–452.

Nissen, E. et al. (1996). Different patterns of oxytocin, prolactin but not cortisol release during breastfeeding in women delivered by caesarean section or by the vaginal route. *Early Human Development*, 45, 103–18.

Nissen, E. et al. (1998). Oxytocin, prolactin, milk production and their relationship with personality traits in women after vaginal delivery or Cesarean section. *Journal of Psychosomatic Obstetrica & Gynecology*, 19, 49–58.

Nowak, R. et al. (1997). Cholecystokinin receptors mediate the development of a preference for the mother by newly born lambs. *Behavior & Neuroscience*, 111, 1375–82.

Nowak, R. et al. (1997). Development of a preferential relationship with the mother by the newborn lamb: importance of the sucking activity. *Physiological Behavior*, 62, 681–8.

Numan, M. (2006). Hypothalamic neural circuits regulating maternal responsiveness toward infants. *Behavioral and Cognitive Neuroscience Review*, 5, 163–90.

Numan M. & Stolzenberg, D. S. Medial preoptic area interactions with dopamine neural systems in the control of the onset and maintenance of maternal behavior in rats. *Frontiers in Neuroendocrinology*, 30, 46–64.

Pedersen, C. A. et al. (1982). Oxytocin induced maternal behaviour in virgin maternal rats. *Science*, 216, 648–649.

Ransjö-Arvidson, A. B. et al. (2001). Maternal analgesia during labor disturbs newborn behavior: effects on breastfeeding, temperature, and crying. *Birth*, 28, 5–12.

Russell, J. A., Leng, G. & Douglas, A. J. (2003). The magnocellular oxytocin system, the fount of maternity: adaptations in pregnancy. *Frontiers in Neuroendocrinology*, 24, 27–61.

Silber, M., Larsson, B. & Uvnäs Moberg, K. (1991). Oxytocin, somatostatin, insulin and gastrin concentrations vis-à-vis late pregnancy, breastfeeding and oral contraceptives. *Acta Obstetricia et Gynecologica Scandinavica*, 70, 283–289.

Stuebe, A. M. et al. (2005). Duration of lactation and incidence of type 2 diabetes. *JAMA*, 294, 2601–2610.

Stuebe, A. M. et al. (2009). Duration of lactation and incidence of myocardial infarction in middle to late adulthood. *American Journal of Obstetrics & Gynecology*, 200, 119–120.

Tops, M. et al. (2007). Anxiety, cortisol, and attachment predict plasma oxytocin. *Psychophysiology*, 44, 444–449.

Uvnäs Moberg, K. (1996). Neuroendocrinology of the mother–child interaction. *Trends in Endocrinology and Metabolism*, 7, 126–31.

Uvnäs Moberg, K. (2006). The role of oxytocin in the development of attachment and maternal adaptations during the postpartum period. In K. H. Brisch & T. Hellbrügge (eds.) *Die Anfänge der Eltern-Kind-Bindung*. Stuttgart: Klett-Cotta.

Widström, A. M. et al. (1987). Gastric suction in healthy newborn infants. Effects on circulation and developing feeding behaviour. *Acta Paediatrica Scandinavica*, 76, 566–72.

6. Oxytocin in adult relationships

Anderson-Hunt, M. & Dennerstein L. (1995). Oxytocin and female sexuality. *Gynecologic and Obstetric Investigation*, 40, 217–221.

Bartels, A. & Zeki, S. (2004). The neural correlates of maternal and romantic love. *Neuroimage*, 21, 1155–1166.

Baumgartner, T. et al. (2008). Oxytocin shapes the neural circuitry of trust and trust adaptation in humans. *Neuron*, 58, 639–50.

Bielsky, I. F. & Young, L. J. (2004). Oxytocin, vasopressin, and social recognition in mammals. *Peptides*, 25, 1565–74.

Blom, M. et al. (2003). Social relations in women with coronary heart disease: the effects of work and marital stress. *Journal of Cardiovascular Risk*, 10, 201–206.

Broad, K. D., Curley, J. P. & Keverne, E. B. (2006). Mother–infant bonding and the evolution of mammalian social relationships. *Philosophical Transactions of the Royal Society B: Biological Sciences*, 29, 2199–214.

Carmichael, M. S. et al. (1987). Plasma oxytocin increases in the human sexual response. *Journal of Clinical Endocrinology and Metabolism*, 64, 27–31.

Ditzen, B. et al. (2008). Intranasal oxytocin increases positive communication and reduces cortisol levels during couple conflict. *Biological Psychiatry*, 65, 728–731.

Domes, G. et al. (2007). Oxytocin attenuates amygdala responses to emotional faces regardless of valence. *Biological Psychiatry*, 62, 1187–1190.

Domes, G. et al. (2007). Oxytocin improves "mind-reading" in humans. *Biological Psychiatry*, 61, 731–733.

Gordon, I. et al. (2008). Oxytocin and cortisol in romantically unattached young adults: associations with bonding and psychological distress. *Psychophysiology*, 45, 349–352.

Guastella, A. J., Mitchell, P. B. & Dadds, M.R. (2008). Oxytocin increases gaze to the eye region of human faces. *Biological Psychiatry*, 63, 3–5.

Heinrichs, M. et al. (2003). Social support and oxytocin interact to suppress cortisol and subjective responses to psychosocial stress. *Biological Psychiatry*, 54, 1389–98.

Heinrichs, M. & Domes, G. (2008). Neuropeptides and social behaviour: effects of oxytocin and vasopressin in humans. *Progress in Brain Research*, 170, 337–350.

Hollander, E. et al. (2007). Oxytocin increases retention of social cognition in autism. *Biological Psychiatry*, 15, 498–503.

Holt-Lunstad, J., Birmingham, W. A. & Light, K. C. (2008). Influence of a "warm touch" support enhancement intervention among married couples on ambulatory blood pressure, oxytocin, alpha amylase, and cortisol. *Psychosomatic Medicine*, 70, 976–985.

Insel, T. R. (2003). Is social attachment an addictive disorder? *Physiological Behavior*, 79, 351–357.

Ishak, W. W., Berman, D. S. & Peters, A. (2008). Male anorgasmia treated with oxytocin. *Journal of Sexual Medicine*, 5, 1022–1024.

Kirsch, P. et al. (2005). Oxytocin modulates neural circuitry for social cognition and fear in humans. *Journal of Neuroscience*, 25, 11489–11493.

Komisaruk, B. R. & Whipple, B. (1998). Love as sensory stimulation: physiological consequences of its deprivation and expression. *Psychoneuroendocrinology*, 23, 927–44.

Kosfeld, M. et al. (2005). Oxytocin increases trust in humans. *Nature*, 435, 673–676.

Krüger, T. H. et al. (2003). Specificity of the neuroendocrine response to orgasm during sexual arousal in men. *Journal of Endocrinology*, 177, 57–64.

Landgraf, R. et al. (2003). Viral vector-mediated gene transfer of the vole V1a vasopressin receptor in the rat septum: improved social discrimination and active social behaviour. *European Journal of Neuroscience*, 18, 403–11.

Light, K. C., Grewen, K. M. & Amico, J. A. (2005). More frequent partner hugs and higher oxytocin levels are linked to lower blood pressure and heart rate in premenopausal women. *Biological Psychology*, 69, 5–21.

Marazziti, D. & Canale, D. (2004). Hormonal changes when falling in love. *Psychoneuroendocrinology*, 29, 931–936.

Martel, F. L. et al. (1993). Opioid receptor blockade reduces maternal affect and social grooming in rhesus monkeys. *Psychoneuroendocrinology*, 18, 307–21.

Martel, F. L. et al. (1995). Effects of opioid receptor blockade on the social behavior of rhesus monkeys living in large family groups. *Developmental Psychobiology*, 28, 71–84.

Neumann, I. D. (2008). Brain oxytocin: a key regulator of emotional and social behaviours in both females and males. *Journal of Neuroendocrinology*, 20, 858–65.

Petrovic, P. et al. (2008). Oxytocin attenuates affective evaluations of conditioned faces and amygdala activity. *Journal of Neuroscience*, 28, 6607–15.

Swain, J. et al. (2007). Brain basis of early parent–infant interactions: psychology, physiology and in vivo functional neuroimaging studies. *Journal of Child Psychology and Psychiatry*, 48, 262–287.

Waldherr, M. & Neumann, I. D. (2007). Centrally released oxytocin mediates mating-induced anxiolysis in male rats. *Proceedings of the National Academy of Sciences of the United States of America*, 104, 16681–4.

Williams, J. R. et al. (1994). Oxytocin administered centrally facilitates formation of a partner preference in female prairie voles (Microtus ochrogaster). *Journal of Neuroendocrinology*, 6, 247–50.

Winslow, J. T. et al. (1993). A role for central vasopressin in pair bonding in monogamous prairie voles. *Nature*, 365, 545–8.

Zak, P. J. (2008). The neurobiology of trust. *Scientific American*, 298, 88–92.

Zak, P. J. & Fakhar, A. (2006). Neuroactive hormones and interpersonal trust: international evidence. *Economics and Human Biology*, 4, 412–29.

Zak, P. J., Kurzban, R. & Matzner, W. T. (2005). Oxytocin is associated with human trustworthiness. *Hormones & Behavior*, 48, 522–527.

Zak, P. J., Stanton, A. A. & Ahmadi, S. (2007). Oxytocin increases generosity in humans. *PLoS ONE*, 2, e1128.

Zeki, S. (2007). The neurobiology of love. *FEBS Letters*, 581, 2575–2579.

Ågren, G. et al. (1997). Olfactory cues from an oxytocin-injected male rat can reduce energy loss in its cagemates. *Neuroreport*, 28, 2551–5.

Ågren, G., Uvnäs Moberg, K. & Lundeberg, T. (1997). Olfactory cues from an oxytocin-injected male rat can induce anti-nociception in its cagemates. *Neuroreport*, 29, 3073–6.

7. Oxytocin and trust

Bartels, A. & Zeki, S. (2004). The neural correlates of maternal and romantic love. *Neuroimage*, 21, 1155–1166.

Baumgartner, T. et al. (2008). Oxytocin shapes the neural circuitry of trust and trust adaptation in humans. *Neuron*, 58, 639–50.

Campbell, D. et al. (2006). A randomized control trial of continuous support in labor by a lay doula. *Journal of Obstetric, Gynecologic and Neonatal Nursing*, 35, 456–64.

Campbell, D. et al. (2007). Female relatives or friends trained as labor doulas: outcomes at 6 to 8 weeks postpartum. *Birth*, 34, 220–227.

Kennell, J. H. & Klaus, M. H. (1998). Bonding: recent observations that alter perinatal care. *Pediatric Review*, 19, 4–12.

Klaus, M. (1998). Mother and infant: early emotional ties. *Pediatrics*, 102, 1244–1246.

Klaus, M. & Kennell, J. H. (1997). The doula: an essential ingredient of childbirth rediscovered. *Acta Paediatrica*, 86, 1034–1036.

Kosfeld, M. et al. (2005). Oxytocin increases trust in humans. *Nature*, 435, 673–676.

McGrath, S. K. & Kennell, J. H. (2008). A randomized controlled trial of continuous labor support for middle-class couples: effect on cesarean delivery rates. *Birth*, 35, 92–7.

Petrovic, P. et al. (2002). Placebo and opioid analgesia-imaging a shared neuronal network. *Science*, 295, 1737–40.

Petrovic, P. et al. (2005). Placebo in emotional processing–induced expectations of anxiety relief activate a generalized modulatory network. *Neuron*, 46, 957–69.

Schore, A. N. (2005). Back to basics: attachment, affect regulation, and the developing right brain: linking developmental neuroscience to pediatrics. *Pediatric Review*, 2, 204–217.

Scott, K. D., Klaus, P. H. & Klaus, M. H. (1999). The obstetrical and postpartum benefits of continuous support during childbirth. *Journal of Women's Health and Gender Based Medicine*, 8, 1257–1264.

Singh, S. & Ernst, E. (2008). *Trick or Treatment? Alternative Medicine on Trial*. Corgi.

Svedman, P., Ingvar, M. & Gordh, T. (2005). "Anxiebo", placebo, and postoperative pain. *BMC Anesthesiology*, 27, 5–9.

Uvnäs Moberg, K., Arn, I. & Magnusson, D. (2005). The psychobiology of emotion: the role of the oxytocinergic system. *International Journal of Behavioral Medicine*, 12, 59–65.

Zak, P. J. (2008). The neurobiology of trust. *Scientific American*, 298, 88–92.

Zak, P. J. & Fakhar, A. (2006). Neuroactive hormones and interpersonal trust: international evidence. *Economics and Human Biology*, 4, 412–29.

Zak, P. J., Kurzban, R. & Matzner, W. T. (2005). Oxytocin is associated with human trustworthiness. *Hormones & Behavior*, 48, 522–527.

Zak, P. J., Stanton, A. A. & Ahmadi, S. (2007). Oxytocin increases generosity in humans. *PLoS ONE*, 2, e1128.

Zeki, S. (2007). The neurobiology of love. *FEBS Letters*, 581, 2575–2579.

8. When closeness is replaced by nutrients

Björkstrand, E. et al. (1996). The oxytocin receptor antagonist 1-deamino-2-D-Tyr-(OEt)-4-Thr-8-Orn-oxytocin inhibits effects of the 5-HT1A receptor agonist 8-OH-DPAT on plasma levels of insulin, cholecystokinin and somatostatin. *Regulatory Peptides*, 63, 47–52.

Eriksson, M. et al. (1994). Role of vagal nerve activity during suckling. Effects on plasma levels of oxytocin, prolactin, VIP, somatostatin, insulin, glucagon, glucose and of milk secretion in lactating rats. *Acta Physiologica Scandinavica*, 151, 453–459.

Feldman, R. et al. (2007). Evidence for a neuroendocrinological foundation of human affiliation: plasma oxytocin levels across pregnancy and the postpartum period predict mother–infant bonding. *Psychological Science*, 18, 965–970.

Harlow, H. F. (1958). The nature of love. *American Psychologist*, 13, 673–685.

Harlow, H. F. & Zimmermann, R. R. (1958). The development of affectional responses in infant monkeys. *Proceedings of the American Philosophical Society*, 102, 501–509.

Holst, S. et al. (2005). Massage-like stroking influences plasma levels of gastrointestinal hormones, including insulin, and increases weight gain in male rats. *Autonomic Neuroscience*, 120, 73–9.

Montagu, A. (1986). *Touching: The human significance of the skin* (3rd edition). New York: Harper and Row.

Nissen, E. et al. (1998). Oxytocin, prolactin, milk production and their relationship with personality traits in women after vaginal delivery or Cesarean section. *Journal of Psychosomatic Obstetrica & Gynecology*, 19, 49–58.

Nowak, R. et al. (1997). Cholecystokinin receptors mediate the development of a preference for the mother by newly born lambs. *Behavior & Neuroscience*, 111, 1375–82.

Nowak, R. et al. (1997). Development of a preferential relationship with the mother by the newborn lamb: importance of the sucking activity. *Physiology & Behavior*, 62, 681–8.

Petersson, M. et al. (1999). Long-term changes in gastrin, cholecystokinin and insulin in response to oxytocin treatment. *Neuroendocrinology*, 69, 202–208.

Törnhage, C. J. et al. (1998). Plasma somatostatin and cholecystokinin levels in preterm infants during kangaroo care with and without nasogastric tube-feeding. *Journal of Pediatric Endocrinology and Metabolism*, 11, 645–651.

Uvnäs Moberg, K. (1989). The gastrointestinal tract in growth and reproduction. *Scientific American*, 261, 78–83.

Uvnäs Moberg, K. (1994). Role of efferent and afferent vagal nerve activity during reproduction: integrating function of oxytocin on metabolism and behaviour. *Psychoneuroendocrinology*, 19, 687–695.

Uvnäs Moberg, K. (2004). Massage and wellbeing, and integrative role for oxytocin? In T. Field (ed.) *Touch in labour and infancy*. J&J Publishing.

Uvnäs Moberg, K. et al. (1987). Release of GI hormones in mother and infant by sensory stimulation. *Acta Paediatrica Scandinavica*, 76, 851–860.

Uvnäs Moberg, K. & Winberg, J. (1989). Role for sensory stimulation in energy economy of the mother and infant with particular regard to the gastrointestinal endocrine system. In E. Lebenthal (ed.) *Textbook of gastroenterology and nutrition in infancy*, 53–62. New York: Raven Press.

Widström, A. M. et al. (1988). Nonnutritive sucking in tube-fed preterm infants: effects on gastric motility and gastric contents of somatostatin. *Journal of Pediatric Gastroenterology and Nutrition*, 7, 517–23.

Widström, A. M. et al. (1989). Maternal somatostatin levels and their correlation with infant birth weight. *Early Human Development*, 20, 165–174.

Widström, A. M. et al. (1990). Short-term effects of early suckling and touch of the nipple on maternal behaviour. *Early Human Development*, 21, 153–63.

9. Closeness provides good health and a longer life

Allen, K. et al. (2002). Cardiovascular reactivity and the presence of pets, friends, and spouses: the truth about cats and dogs. *Psychosomatic Medicine*, 64, 727–39.

Berget, B., Ekeberg, O. & Braastad, B. O. (2008). Animal-assisted therapy with farm animals for persons with psychiatric disorders: effects on self-efficacy, coping ability and quality of life, a randomized controlled trial. *Clinical Practice and Epidemiology in Mental Health*, 11, 4–9.

Blom, M. et al. (2003). Social relations in women with coronary heart disease: the effects of work and marital stress. *Journal of Cardiovascular Risk*, 10, 201–206.

Castelli, P., Hart, L. A. & Zasloff, R. L. (2001). Companion cats and the social support systems of men with AIDS. *Psychological Reports*, 89, 177–187.

DeVries, A. C., Glasper, E. R. & Detillion, C. E. (2003). Social modulation of stress responses. *Physiological Behavior*, 79, 399–407.

Diego, M. A. & Field, T. (2009). Moderate pressure massage elicits a parasympathetic nervous system response. *International Journal of Neuroscience*, 119, 630–638.

Diego, M. A. et al. (2007). Preterm infant massage elicits consistent increases in vagal activity and gastric motility that are associated with greater weight gain. *Acta Paediatrica*, 96, 1588–1591.

Field, T. et al. (2002). Fibromyalgia pain and substance P decrease and sleep improves after massage therapy. *Journal of Clinical Rheumatology*, 8, 72–76.

Field, T. et al. (2008). Massage therapy reduces pain in pregnant women, alleviates prenatal depression in both parents and improves their relationships. *Journal of Bodywork and Movement Therapies*, 12, 146–150.

Friedmann, E. & Thomas, S. A. (1995). Pet ownership, social support, and one-year survival after acute myocardial infarction in the Cardiac Arrhythmia Suppression Trial (CAST). *American Journal of Cardiology*, 76, 1213–1217.

Güçlü, B. et al. (2007). Tactile sensitivity of normal and autistic children. *Somatosensory and Motor Research*, 24, 21–33.

Hernandez-Reif, M., Diego, M. & Field, T. (2007). Preterm infants show reduced stress behaviors and activity after 5 days of massage therapy. *Infant Behavior and Development*, 30, 557–61.

Holt-Lunstad, J., Birmingham, W. A. & Light, K. C. (2008). Influence of a "warm touch" support enhancement intervention among married couples on ambulatory blood pressure, oxytocin, alpha amylase, and cortisol. *Psychosomatic Medicine*, 70, 976–985.

Kern, J. K. et al. (2007). Sensory correlations in autism. *Autism*, 11, 123–34.

Kosfeld, M. et al. (2005). Oxytocin increases trust in humans. *Nature*, 435, 673–676.

Light, K. C. et al. (2005). Oxytocinergic activity is linked to lower blood pressure and vascular resistance during stress in postmenopausal women on estrogen replacement. *Hormones and Behavior*, 47, 540–8.

Light, K. C., Grewen, K. M. & Amico, J. A. (2005). More frequent partner hugs and higher oxytocin levels are linked to lower blood pressure and

heart rate in premenopausal women. *Biological Psychology*, 69, 5–21.
Odendaal, J. S. & Meintjes, R. A. (2003). Neurophysiological correlates of affiliative behavior between humans and dogs. *The Veterinary Journal*, 165, 296–301.
Ornish, D. (1998). *Love and survival. The scientific basis for the healing power of intimacy*. London: Harper Collins.
Paredes, J. et al. (2006). Social experience influences hypothalamic oxytocin in the WHHL rabbit. *Psychoneuroendocrinology*, 31, 1062–1075.
Raina, P. et al. (1999). Influence of companion animals on the physical and psychological health of older people: an analysis of a one-year longitudinal study. *Journal of the American Geriatric Society*, 47, 323–9.
Robb, S. S. & Stegman, C. E. (1983). Companion animals and elderly people: a challenge for evaluators of social support. *Gerontologist*, 23, 277–282.
Rosengren, A., Wilhelmsen, L. & Orth-Gomér, K. (2004). Coronary disease in relation to social support and social class in Swedish men. A 15 year follow-up in the study of men born in 1933. *European Heart Journal*, 25, 56–63.
Sachser, N., Durschlag, M. & Hirzel, D. (1998). Social relationships and the management of stress. *Psychoneuroendocrinology*, 23, 891–904.
Singh, S. & Ernst, E. (2008). *Trick or Treatment? Alternative Medicine on Trial*. Corgi.
Szeto, A. et al. (2008). Oxytocin attenuates NADPH-dependent superoxide activity and IL-6 secretion in macrophages and vascular cells. *American Journal of Physiology: Endocrinology and Metabolism*, 295, 1495–501.
Uvnäs Moberg, K. (1997). Physiological and endocrine effects of social contact. *Annals of the New York Academy of Science*, 807, 146–63.
Uvnäs Moberg, K. (1998). Oxytocin may mediate the benefits of positive social interaction and emotions. *Psychoneuroendocrinology*, 23, 819–35. Review.
Uvnäs Moberg, K. et al. (2001). Oxytocin facilitates behavioural, metabolic and physiological adaptations during lactation. *Applied Animal Behavior Science*, 72, 225–234.
Uvnäs Moberg, K. & Petersson, M. (2005). Antistress, känsla, empati och socialt stöd. In R. Ekman & B. Arnetz (ed.) *Från molekyl till individ*. Stockholm: Liber.
Uvnäs Moberg, K. & Petersson, M. (2008). Molecular anti-stress systems. In B. Arnetz & R. Ekman (eds.) *Stress sculpturing the brain to health or disease*. New York: Wiley Press.
Von Knorring, A.-L. et al. (2008). Massage decreases aggression in preschool children: a long-term study. *Acta Paediatrica*, 97, 1265–1269.
Wang, H. X., Mittleman, M. A. & Orth-Gomér, K. (2005). Influence of social support on progression of coronary artery disease in women. *Social Science & Medicine*, 60, 599–607.
Zak, P. J., Kurzban, R. & Matzner, W. T. (2005). Oxytocin is associated with human trustworthiness. *Hormones & Behavior*, 48, 522–527.
Zak, P. J., Stanton, A. A. & Ahmadi, S. (2007). Oxytocin increases generosity in humans. *PLoS ONE*, 2, e1128.

10. The oxytocin heritage

Boucher, M. et al. (2004). Comparison of carbetocin and oxytocin for the prevention of postpartum hemorrhage following vaginal delivery: a double-blind randomized trial. *International Journal of Gynecology and Obstetrics*, 26, 481–488.

Burnham, T. C. (2007). High-testosterone men reject low ultimatum game offers. *Proceedings of the Royal Society: Biological Science*, 274, 2327–2330.

Bystrova, K. et al. (2009). Early contact versus separation: Effects on mother–infant interaction one year later. *Birth*, 36, 97–109.

Caldwell, H. K., Stephens, S. L. & Young, W. S. III (2008). Oxytocin as a natural antipsychotic: a study using oxytocin knockout mice. *Molecular Psychiatry*, 14, 190–196.

Ditzen, B. et al. (2008). Intranasal oxytocin increases positive communication and reduces cortisol levels during couple conflict. *Biological Psychiatry*, 65, 728–731.

Grape, C. et al. (2003). Does singing promote well-being?: An empirical study of professional and amateur singers during a singing lesson. *Integrative Physiological and Behavioral Science*, 38, 65–74.

Hegner, P. (2008). *Leken som berör; sagor, lekar, sånger och ramsor till massage*. Stockholm: Natur & Kultur.

Heinrichs, M. & Gaab, J. (2007). Neuroendocrine mechanisms of stress and social interaction: implications for mental disorders. *Current Opinion in Psychiatry*, 20, 158–62.

Hollander, E. et al. (2003). Oxytocin infusion reduces repetitive behaviors in adults with autistic and Asperger's disorders. *Neuropsychopharmacology*, 28, 193–198.

Hollander, E. et al. (2007). Oxytocin increases retention of social cognition in autism. *Biological Psychiatry*, 15, 498–503.

Huotari, A. & Herzig, K. H. (2008). Vitamin D and living in northern latitudes – an endemic risk area for vitamin D deficiency. *International Journal of Circumpolar Health*, 67, 164–178.

Insel, T. R. (2003). Is social attachment an addictive disorder? *Physiological Behavior*, 79, 351–357.

Marazziti, D. & Catena Dell'osso, M. (2008). The role of oxytocin in neuropsychiatric disorders. *Current Medicinal Chemistry*, 15, 698–704.

Odent, M. (2007). When love hormones become useless. *Midwifery Today with International Midwife*, 22, 66.

Ohlsson, B. et al. (2005). Effects of long-term treatment with oxytocin in chronic constipation; a doubleblind, placebo-controlled pilot trial. *Neurogastroenterology and Motility*, 17, 697–704.

Raina, P. et al. (1999). Influence of companion animals on the physical and psychological health of older people: an analysis of a one-year longitudinal study. *Journal of the American Geriatric Society*, 47, 323–9.

Robb, S. S. & Stegman, C. E. (1983). Companion animals and elderly people: a challenge for evaluators of social support. *Gerontologist*, 23, 277–282.

Thompson, M. R. et al. (2007). A role for oxytocin and 5-HT(1A) receptors in the prosocial effects of 3,4methylenedioxymethamphetamine ("ecstasy"). *Neuroscience*, 146, 509–14.

Uvnäs Moberg, K. et al. (1999). Oxytocin as a possible mediator of SSRI-induced antidepressant effects. *Psychopharmacology*, 142, 95–101.

Uvnäs Moberg, K., Alster, P. & Svensson, T. H. (1992). Amperozide and clozapine but not haloperidol or raclopride increase the secretion of oxytocin in rats. *Psychopharmacology*, 109, 473–476.

Uvnäs Moberg, K. & Petersson, M. (2004). Oxytocin–biochemical link for human relations. Mediator of antistress, well-being, social interaction, growth, healing. *Läkartidningen*, 101, 2634–2639.

Uvnäs Moberg, K. & Petersson, M. (2005). Oxytocin, a mediator of anti-stress, well-being, social interaction, growth and Healing. *Zeitschrift für Psychosomatische Medizin und Psychotherapie*, 51, 57–80.

Uvnäs Moberg, K. & Petersson, M. (2009). Role of oxytocin and oxytocin related effects in manual therapies. In H. H. King, W. Jänig & P. H. Patterson (eds.) *The science and clinical application of manual therapy*. Elsevier.

Zak, P. J. (2004). Neuroeconomics. *Philosophical Transactions of the Royal Society B: Biological Science*, 359, 1737–1748.

Zak, P. J. (2008). The neurobiology of trust. *Scientific American*, 298, 88–92.

Zak, P. J. & Fakhar, A. (2006). Neuroactive hormones and interpersonal trust: international evidence. *Economics and Human Biology*, 4, 412–29.

Zak, P. J., Kurzban, R. & Matzner, W. T. (2005). Oxytocin is associated with human trustworthiness. *Hormones & Behavior*, 48, 522–527.

Zak, P. J., Stanton, A. A. & Ahmadi, S. (2007). Oxytocin increases generosity in humans. *PLoS ONE*, 2, e1128.

Index

Pinter & Martin (www.pinterandmartin.com) is an independent book publisher based in London, with distribution throughout the world. We specialise in psychology, pregnancy, birth and parenting, fiction and yoga, and publish authors who challenge the status quo, such as Elliot Aronson, Grantly Dick-Read, Ina May Gaskin, Stanley Milgram, Guillermo O'Joyce, Michel Odent, Gabrielle Palmer, Stuart Sutherland and Frank Zappa.

Doula UK (www.doula.org.uk) was set up in 2001 to provide a network for doulas and is the largest organisation of doulas in Great Britain. There are currently over 550 members all of whom adhere to a Code of Conduct and have trained through an organisation who follow the Doula UK Core Curriculum for Doula Preparation. The not-for-profit organisation has a 'Find a Doula' facility to enable parents to find doula support in their area.